YOU CAN *live* WITHOUT A PANCREAS

YOU CAN *live* WITHOUT A PANCREAS

CLYDE VAUGHAN
SHIRLEY VAUGHAN

TATE PUBLISHING
AND ENTERPRISES, LLC

Published by Tate Publishing & Enterprises, LLC
127 E. Trade Center Terrace | Mustang, Oklahoma 73064 USA
1.888.361.9473 | www.tatepublishing.com

Tate Publishing is committed to excellence in the publishing industry. The company reflects the philosophy established by the founders, based on Psalm 68:11,
"The Lord gave the word and great was the company of those who published it."

Book design copyright © 2012 by Tate Publishing, LLC. All rights reserved.
Cover design by Kristen Verser
Interior design by Chelsea Womble

Published in the United States of America

ISBN: 978-1-62024-374-9
1. Medical / General
2. Biography & Autobiography / Medical
12.05.18

To my wife and angel, Shirley, with all my love

TABLE OF CONTENTS

INTRODUCTION:
Why Did We Write This Book?

You are holding in your hands the book we wish we read before we began our adventures in surviving modern medicine, chemicals and food without my pancreas. Growing up and then raising a family in rural southeastern Virginia, Shirley and I have seen up close what everyone else on the planet has noticed: Life has changed in fundamental ways we couldn't imagine fifty or even five years ago. While advances in medicine, chemical and food production continue to impress us all, there comes a point in everyone's life when you realize that much of the machinery of these industrial systems are running ahead with no thought and little care for the humans they were intended to serve. In fact, they feed on each other, as the chemicals in our environment and processed foods in our diets lead us to chronic diseases, pharmaceuticals and hospital stays that feed the broken health care system, which in turn, shoots us back out into the world with little guidance on what health is and back to the cycle of noxious food and chemical overload. Everybody wins on the corporate end, just not regular people trying to have healthy, normal lives. Maybe, like us, you won't give much attention to this truth until you lose a vital organ, like I did, or suffer from one of the many skyrocketing chronic diseases in the epidemic accompanying all this industrial "progress".

After I lost my pancreas to an emergency total pancreatectomy, TP, and began living as an ongoing medical experiment in 2004, my life depended upon unraveling the grandiose promises of modern medicine, chemicals and food. The hospital-contracted infection that annihilated my pancreas (our bodies' source of insulin and digestive enzymes) and left me a "beyond brittle" diabetic at least did not kill me, as it does 99,000 people a year in the United States. [1] (Two million people a year contract hospital-borne infections a year, according to the CDC.)

From the beginning, my doctors told Shirley and I they had little guidance for how I was to live without this vital organ. While an Internet search today shows a handful of people, such as Betsy Hilfiger (the designer Tommy's sister), are living without a pancreas, no books or how-to guides were around then or now. Thanks to a Johns Hopkins online message board, during the writing of this book I found a small, self-run support group of TP survivors on a Yahoogroups' discussion board. The discussion board listed around 70 members, but only around a dozen were active posters with six to 50 messages a month.

The Yahoogroup participants were generous in their support for this book and in sharing their experiences. In a poll and during individual interviews, the active posters shared with us their lack of medical preparation for living without their pancreases, and some, years later, were still suffering. A few emailed us back personally and said they were reluctant to share their suffering openly on the message board because they did not want to discourage others. A few also said they survived their TPs with no problem. While everyone's personal story of how they arrived at the decision to have a TP – either facing cancer or pancreatitis — is different, our stories were the same on the other side of losing our pancreases: We were all beyond brittle diabetics struggling with a stratospheric learning curve for the first few years.

As one group member, Jonathan Lightman from Carmichael, Calif., stated, "My wife, Janice, and I both believe you have to be brilliant to survive the recovery from a TP, to figure it all out for yourself." Another member observed, "If you came into your TP through pancreatitis, you are probably still in pain and wondering if the surgery was the right thing to do. If you came into your TP through cancer, you are just grateful to be alive."

Some of the group members took part in groundbreaking surgical techniques, with the Da Vinci robot, or with the early detection offered by a Familial Tumor Registry, genetic screening and CAPS, cancer of the pancreas screening programs. Ted Levy shared that his TP and follow-up medical care were with Johns Hopkins, "the crème de la crème of medical care."

"Everyone in the group survey said they did not get enough information to handle the diabetes, I will say no as well, despite being treated at Johns Hopkins and being surrounded by the best resources in the country or the world," Levy said. "Even though I have great medical care and my doctors are great, even though it is a group of endocrinologists, they have very little experience with someone who has had a TP. Their experience is usually with people who are dying. That is why our Yahoogroup is for post-TP-diabetics, because everyone has the experience of losing the pancreas and becoming brittle diabetics."

Another shared experience of the group was constantly correcting *doctors* who told them, during their aftercare, that they couldn't live without a pancreas. Lightman, who is a lobbyist, said he grew so tired of correcting doctors that he began to quip, "Oh, did I say I had my pancreas removed? I meant to say I had pancakes for breakfast." The ignorance of doctors, much less the public, that there are pancreatitis and cancer survivors living without their pancreases is not surprising. The small group of TP survivors huddled together on an internet island did not amount to a large enough sample to make the radar of the medical establishment. CDC, the US Centers for Disease Control and Prevention, told us they do not have statistics on TPs because they are too rare. Ditto with the National Center for Health Statistics. [2]

Amazingly, as this book was being written, a new study advocating TPs, dated May 20, 2010, appeared on the Web site for PubMed, a reliable source of medical study information and a service of the U.S. National Library of Medicine and the National Institutes of Health. The free online databse, at www.pubmed. gov, comprises more than 19 million citations for biomedical literature from MEDLINE, life science journals, and online books.

The new study examined 65 total pancreatectomies between 1996 and 2008, both elective and non-elective. The study, conducted by the University of Verona, Italy, explained, "Total Pancreatectomy (TP) has been performed rarely in the past because of its high morbidity and mortality. Because outcomes of pancreatic surgery as well as management of pancreatic insufficiency have improved markedly, enthusiasm for TP has increased." The study concluded that, "TP can be performed safely with no mortality and acceptable morbidity. Postoperative pancreatic insufficiency can be managed safely... TP is an effective operation in selected patients." [3]

No other current American studies or universities expand on this possibility. And we polled American universities and hospitals, both by phone and email through their media departments, to ask for help gathering individual hospital statistics since the national centers did not track or maintain statistics on TPs. Every university hospital media officer stated they did not or could not give us this information, though many were nice and wished us well on our search.

We stopped asking for statistics and started asking if it was possible for a recommendation for TPs to be forthcoming from an official medical authority. A volunteer with the American Pancreatic Association told us it would depend upon who we asked as to what opinion we would get on the possibility of TPs eventually becoming recommended and mainstreamed.

If total pancreatectomies are offered in the future as an alternative treatment for patients who may otherwise have suffered or died from cancer or pancreatic diseases, we are happy to have taken the time to share our story with those who will want to know what they could be facing. Our story is certainly not everyone's story. In fact, we found no one who had lost their pancreas to hospital-acquired infection. And we sincerely hope no one goes through the trials we faced in 2004 and over those first years. But one aspect of our story *was* echoed repeatedly through the Yahoogroup TP survivors: Minimal or no medical preparation and guidance after a TP equaled years of horrific stress on our bodies and families until everyone "figured it out" for themselves. The real tragedy is the one that will never be told. With no tracking of this rare surgery, how would we ever know who didn't "figure it out" in time?

Shirley and I wrote this book together to share with you our personal story and our discoveries about living a healthy and sane life in our radically changed and changing world. We found out modern medicine is not the "cure" we were raised to believe it to be and wished it could be. It really only works when we, as patients, take full responsibility for our health, even in the midst of severe illness. Modern food is mostly dead, chemically-processed gut wad that is now scientifically linked to chronic diseases, such as diabetes and pancreatic cancer specifically (through high fructose corn syrup according to a 2010 UCLA study).[4] And our homes and neighborhoods can be minefields of chemical toxins for those living with immune-system challenges from chronic diseases.

While I was motivated to investigate the truth of modern medicine, chemicals and food because I became a "beyond brittle" diabetic after losing my pancreas, you may eventually be forced to do the same for a different reason. Statistically speaking, your chances of ending up diabetic increase every year you are alive. According to the American Diabetes Association, one in 20 Americans can now expect to become diabetic in their lifetime. [5]

While I did not lose my pancreas to cancer, Shirley and I wonder how many people would choose to live without a pancreas if they knew it was an option. As we conducted research for this book, we only found a handful of people — including Betsy Hilfiger, sister of the designer, Tommy — who tested for pre-cancerous cells in her pancreas in 2006 and opted for a prophylactic TP. Her story can be found at the Pancreas Center of Columbia University online. [6]

A few Yahoogroup members, like its moderator Ted Levy, caught their cancers early by participating in CAPS (cancer of the pancreas screening), through the National Familial Pancreas Tumor Registry, established at Johns Hopkins a dozen years ago to track pancreatic cancer patients and their relatives. Levy's father, uncle and cousin died from pancreatic cancer. He believes being a part of the tumor registry and CAPS program saved his life. "I am thankful everyday for my medical care and sympathetic doctors who will look up things for me, but I am one in a hundred," says Levy. "This book is something that needs to be done". His story is featured at the end of this book.

Pancreatic cancer is one of the deadliest types of cancer. Even though it is only the 11th most common cancer in the United States, it is the fourth-leading cause of cancer death, because nearly all the patients die. Every year about 42,470 individuals are diagnosed and 35,240 a year die from the disease, according to the National Cancer Center with the National Institutes of Health (visit them at www.cancer.gov). The prognosis for pancreatic cancer is poor, as less than five percent are still alive five years after diagnosis and complete remission is rare.

Unfortunately, as all of these grim statistics show, Shirley and I have a lot of company on our quest to be an active part of our own health care. In our book, in addition to accompanying us on our journey to wellness, you will find resources for patient advocacy, chemical-free living and growing or finding fresh, local food.

I hope you will be inspired to cherish the people in your life who care for you, as I do my wife, Shirley. Her *Caring for the Caregivers* chapter and its tips is a gift of insight to other family members who may find themselves becoming nurse, researcher, advocate and companion for a chronically ill loved one.

Coming to terms with the loss of my pancreas and my new life as a brittle diabetic felt as if a bomb went off in our lives. As I swam in and out of consciousness that first year, through high and low blood sugar swings and a suicide attempt, it was the face of an angel, my precious wife, Shirley, who ministered to me and kept me alive. Over the coming years, as the smoke continued to clear, we became more aware of and began to believe and trust in the parts that didn't blow up: our love for one another and our children, our common sense and our good, clean food from our own garden. These were the things that really mattered, really nourished our bodies and souls and in the end, really kept us alive. And this – this hard-won wisdom gleaned from surviving and thriving despite the naysayers and the odds — is what we wish to share with you in this book.

We need to also give credit to one other source of our inspiration as survivors. One of many benefits of being rooted for life in the Commonwealth of Virginia, is that we are surrounded by the local, state and national history of our home place that constantly points to the bigger picture: to the relationship between our individual lives and choices and their contributions to our collective community and country. As you will also discover through our story telling, as Virginians, it wasn't hard for us to understand that our troubles and victories with industry-oriented, modern life are not just ours alone or new to this century.

As the son of a tenant farmer, I was raised with a hoe I my hand witnessing the truth of where our food came from – a healthy soil and hard labor. This understanding, of the value of my education as a farmer's son, is a foundation I have returned to for clues to being healthy and surviving as a brittle diabetic. I have company and confirmation on this part of my journey. Many Native American tribes, battling higher than average diabetes rates, have also found wellness in returning to their roots, their "cultural identity" that is also ground in the stories of their family traditions, tribal histories and local foods. [7] Today, our entire nation is remembering what is it to grow "victory gardens" as we did after World War II. And just looking around at the number of our neighbors who have jumped on the national bandwagon of growing at least part of our own food – as most of our grandparents used to do — it is not hard to see that many people are discovering where nourishment for our bodies and souls used to come from, not so long ago. It seems like many of us, whether for health or economic reasons, are making a long-awaited and now necessary return home to our roots.

If our book helps you to find a reason or a way to help yourself survive modern medicine, chemicals and food and live a healthy, loving life, then we could say that our efforts and insights have been worth our long journey.

God Bless you and your families,
Clyde and Shirley Vaughan
April 2011

CHAPTER ONE

How I Lost My Pancreas and With It, Our Dream of Peace

"Love conquers all things; let us too surrender to Love"

—Virgil

During four decades of marriage, with a family of eight, my wife and I regularly jumped into our 1988 Monte Carlo in our small, rural town and onto the shortest escape route — the Jamestown-Scotland ferry, which shuttles folks from our neighboring Surry County to the tourist town of Williamsburg across the James River. On the Surry side of the river — and an hour's drive through farmland dotted with historic markers, Victorian houses and country diners patronized by people who know each other's lineage — is the county where I was born and where Shirley and I raised our six children. On the other side of the twenty-minute ferry ride lies "America's Birthplace", as their slogan says. The tourist version of Historic Jamestowne, is Jamestown Settlement, whose three replica 17th century ships are so close to the ferry landing you can spy the colorful, docked ships, usually full of school children, as you drive over the ferry's clanking exit ramps, past a long line of cars waiting to load, and toward America's colonial capital and the college town of Williamsburg.

Dozens of times over the years, Shirley and I have stood with other passengers on the deck of the two-story ferry and marveled at the developments in Historic Jamestowne. The original landing site of the first 104 English settlers commissioned by the Virginia Company of London on the small island — now a national park – is a separate, sacred site preserved down the river bank from the museum and tourist attraction of "Jamestown Settlement". After much theorizing and exploration, in 1994, archeologists finally located the original, legendary triangular fort partially submerged in the river's edge and began covering parts of the site with blue plastic space-age domes, a stark contrast beside an ancient brick church and a rare view, visible only from the river.

Along the edge of the reconstructed fort's log pole walls stand the haunting brick ruins of the original 1686 church tower. And even though we couldn't see her from the ferry, we knew the slightly larger than life statue of Pocahontas stood just a few feet from the low wrought iron fence protecting the crumbling sarcophagus and headstones in the church's grassy cemetery. Archeological evidence shows Pocahontas' relatives lived near those same river banks for more than 10,000 years before English settlers arrived. While Pocahontas is hidden from ferry passengers, to the naked eye the most imposing structure from the ferry deck is the 103 foot tall Tercentenary obelisk jutting needle-like up and over the church and fort to commemorate the landing of the first colonists and the injection of the New World ideas of progress, efficiency and manifest destiny that would take only 200 years to displace Pocahontas' relatives and 400 years to consume and transform the entire, virgin continent of North America. Of course, there were other ideas introduced to the world through Jamestowne, ideas that were refined in the budding nation's colonial capital buildings of neighboring Williamsburg. Those noble ideas disavowed humans as cogs to serve industrial machinery and its tyrannical dictates and defiantly proclaimed human beings as individuals with rights to freedom and liberty and whose self-determining lives should be served by the products and services of industry.

The ongoing battle for control of the vision of the New World and question of "who serves whom" only escalated and changed forms in 400 years where it is now carried forward through the tenets of "globalization" — accompanied by a chorus of dissenters pointing out the epidemics of chronic diseases, natural resource destruction and pollution left in the wake of modern industrial "progress." The question now is, do industry-modeled businesses, like modern medicine, chemicals and agri-business really serve and support our human needs, or are we here to provide those industrial systems with human fodder for the mechanized mill? How do we find the time and energy in our modern busy lives to ask these questions, much less find out the answers? What happens if people, the possessors of compassion and common sense, don't, won't or can't control the intention and direction of a heartless, mechanical-minded model that shapes our everyday lives and world?

I don't think Shirley and I asked ourselves these questions before 2004. Our perennially broken car radio meant we had lots of time for hypothesizing and envisioning life "back then," but we could not imagine my life was eventually going to depend upon finding the answers to these questions.

After a day of freedom out in the "world" we would return, sated and sleepy, to the ferry docks. On the sunset cruise home, we would float past Jamestowne's darkened banks, exit the Surry-side landing by the steep uphill beach road and wind home spying deer and wild turkeys through quiet byways whose small route number signs would quickly lose a "foreigner" – meaning, anyone not born and raised in these parts.

Our side of the river boasts one of the oldest working plantations in existence, Chippokes, by one of Jamestown's settlers and continuously farmed since 1619 and now a living history exhibit and state park. But there are other sites and stories on our side of the river, right down the street from our Southampton County home, that no one boasts about, stories that make you hold your breath, waiting for a disclaimer that they couldn't possibly be true so you can breathe again.

When reflecting upon the setting and context of our personal lives, what we know is, this part of the world is our home. And all of its rich Virginia beauty goes part and parcel with the ghosts of the past, who will whisper lessons to you if you pause to listen.

We put our hearts into our family home over the years, a modest brick rancher with soaring pines lining the front yard and, in the back, a double mirror image boxwood hedge maze anchored by a 200 year-old popular tree. A large V for Vaughan — drawn with boxwoods — stands at the entrance to the maze. I threw the V in for good measure with the thought of our grandchildren playing hide-and-seek along the paths, which they do. I designed and constructed the maze from 500 seedlings I sprouted myself 25 years earlier from Berkeley Plantation — the Virginia farm that notoriously ousted New England for the site of the First Thanksgiving.

Being a Virginian by birth meant having a historic reference point for every aspect of our lives. Family day trips and extended vacations, as well as mine and Shirley's escapades, were often spent at some historic site or another whose purpose was to remind us of how we and all Americans arrived at this point in our individual and collective histories. Being a Virginian means you were probably raised or oriented to think about things in a long-term, big picture way that not everyone else is these days — a handy skill when you need perspective on the dramas of your own life.

Although our life together had been rationed its own ups and downs, by the time we made it through raising six children and I retired after 40 years as a senior lab analyst with a local chemical company, our dreams and plans for our golden years were firmly in place. We were ready to extend our getaways out into the world beyond day trips across the river. We had taken care of ourselves and were proud that we could still fit into our wedding clothes. We loved our church of more than 40 years, where I sang in the choir. Neither of us had taken up bad habits like smoking or drinking, but stuck to our common sense path to get where we'd been headed for forty years together.

The turn our lives took in the summer of 2004 we had not, and could not, foresee. No one could. The thought that I would become a living medical experiment, and Shirley would become a dozen roles necessary to keep me alive, did not reside even in the periphery of our busy days. The careful planning of our lives, the dutiful execution I gave to my career and Shirley to our home, the thoughtful attention we gave to our bodies, our children, our future, was in preparation for those final years together that we would spend in peace, knowing we had fulfilled our obligations and were now free to enjoy our lives. Peace. That was our dream.

Our dream was still intact in August of 2004, when I held Shirley's hand in our local hospital before being wheeled into the operating room. The long-scheduled gallbladder surgery was a bump in the road, one of many we had weathered, together and apart. We believed one of the first things we would do when I recovered was hop into the Monte Carlo and hit our escape route across the river, with the wind in our hair, not a care in the world, relishing the freedom we had earned.

And then, a microscopic detail altered the future. During the gallbladder surgery, a hospital contagion shimmied up a drain tube implanted in my pancreas. It would be early fall, and three admissions later, by the time Shirley found herself shouting to anyone who would listen in the hospital hallway, demanding the small-town surgeons transfer me to a university center where there were "real" doctors or she and my son were putting me in the car and taking me out of there. By that time, our dream had already disintegrated, along with my pancreas. We just didn't know it.

Looking back, as we have so many times through the fog of the last few years, one thing becomes clear: It was Shirley's secret that kept me alive and salvaged the remnants of our dream.

Shirley's sister says she will never tell their secret. She will never admit the truth of their childhood. Whether Shirley was born with innate survival skills or whether they appeared later in her life, the fact is, in 1945, as American GIs were beginning their long-awaited return home from the European Theater of World War II as seasoned soldiers who had witnessed and survived the hell of war, a seven-year-old Shirley entered an orphanage in North Carolina with her siblings, where she would spend the next ten years of her childhood honing the survival skills necessary to live through a different kind of hell.

She won't tell me, or anyone, the whole truth of their time there. But through fragments and whispers, I have glimpsed a wiry, dark-haired, shoeless Shirley in the orphanage washrooms, ironing mountains of linens with an iron "heavier than she was," she says. Shirley is shoeless in my imaginings of her because the children were not allowed to wear shoes from May until

September. They were only allowed shoes on Saturday evenings to polish for church the next day, and then the shoes were taken away until the next weekend.

Shirley stops and shakes her head when she gets to scenes that she says would make the hair on your head stand straight up. Her harsh childhood did not kill Shirley's spirit. It was a wizened and witty 16-year-old Shirley that walked out the doors of the North Carolina orphanage and into a minister's home with her sister.

"There were mornings when we would hear the matron singing — 'Zippity doo dah, Zippity aye. My, oh my, what a wonderful day!' — and we would cluck our tongues and say to each other, 'Nope, not today'. And set about our plans for entertaining ourselves," laughs Shirley.

The orphanage still exists in Thomasville, North Carolina, and was celebrating their 125th anniversary in 2010. The Baptist Children's home promises hope and healing to families now, but in the dark years following World War II, things were different. When Shirley and I visited the Web site, she couldn't believe the beautiful, comfortable beds and especially the gleaming gymnasium.

"They get to play!" she cried. "We were told that idle hands were the devil's playground and if we had time to play, then we had time to work. This doesn't even look like the same place."

Shirley says she doesn't need to "go there" with the details, "just read Oliver Twist, and you'll get the idea." A picture of Shirley as a child, before entering the orphanage, sits on the bookshelves in our living room. Her brother gave us this picture. In the black and white photo she is wearing a short summer dress and a beaming smile. We have no other pictures from Shirley's childhood.

Through my own insights, gleaned from Shirley's short storytelling and spending more than half of our lives together, I believe

Shirley sharpened two survival skills in particular in her childhood: her acid, quick wit and searing but honest humor. Over
the past six years of coming to grips with the loss of my pancreas
and with it, our dream of peace, it has been Shirley's ability to find
a perspective on anything to help us laugh that has cut through
many a dire situation and released us both from weighty bonds of
depression and hopelessness.

At what point could we have been spared the nightmare that
was coming? The "shoulds" are endless. Should we have not
trusted the surgeon that I knew from a regional choir group?
Should we have Googled every surgical risk known for the common cholecystectomy? Should we have had our children pum-
mel the hospital staff with requests for information on questions
none of knew to ask? Should we have scheduled this common
surgery at a larger, more state of the art facility with university
caliber doctors?

One "should" we could answer was this: A routine gallbladder
removal by a surgeon in a small-town hospital *should* have been
over with in August. Shirley and I *should* have hit the road by the
end of summer. But the surgeon who opened me up and took out
the gallbladder decided to puncture a pseudocyst that had formed
on the neighboring organ, the pancreas, and point a drainage tube
outside a hole in my abdomen before closing me up. Medical
experts testifying in the lawsuit years later would say this grave
error of judgment — to act surgically upon such an "unforgiving"
organ as the pancreas — *should* never have happened.

We knew the baseball-sized pseudocyst was there, as it had
been detected on the head of the pancreas by a CAT scan months
before the gallbladder surgery. The gallbladder surgery was post-
poned until the inflammation cooled. Which it did. So the mystery of why the surgeon decided to act upon the pseudocyst and

violate the pancreas is still a mystery, even after the doctor testi-fied at the medical malpractice court hearing. Even more mysteri-ous and shocking was the surgeon's complete silence on the "gan-grene" he supposedly found in my pancreas during the gallbladder surgery until the day – nearly a month later – that I was finally transferred to a hospital more equipped to handle the emergency surgical removal or "scooping out" of what was left of my pan-creas, as the surgeon at the large, city hospital described to us.

Gangrene? A "charcoal black gangrene", as the local surgeon testified during the court case, though somehow neglected to record in his surgical notes or tell any other hospital doctors while I was lying in a hospital bed for nearly a month. Why was a post-op notation of gangrene or the announcement that I had lost a major organ to anyone never made? Because there was no gangrene or infection of any kind at the time of the gallbladder surgery. That he did write in his surgical notes: no infection. The infection, in reality, came later.

Every time I try to summarize the events that lead to the loss of my pancreas in the summer of 2004, I find my own words too bizarre to be believed. This is why I decided to let you read the surgeon's account of what happened in his own words, taken directly from the court transcript, for yourself. You decide what happened.

In the end, it was the drainage tube the local surgeon inserted into the pseudocyst on the pancreas' head, which he shouldn't have touched, that served as the superhighway for an enterprising hospital germ to set up camp in my pancreas. I, like two million Americans a year, contracted a hospital-born infection. Really, I was lucky. Of the 99,000 patients a year who die from hospital infections, I lived. [1] But only because, after I held Shirley's hand and told her I was sure I was dying, she stomped her foot, shook her hands and yelled to get the attention of the hospital staff and doctors who were never told about the nonexistent "gangrene" by the surgeon, until it came time to finally transfer me to a better hospital.

I did not "lose" my pancreas. I did not choose to have my pancreas removed. It rotted away from a post-surgical hospital infection while still lying in my abdomen as I lay in a hospital bed surrounded by medical staff for three weeks in the late summer of 2004. By the time the doctors and staff took Shirley's foot stamping dance seriously, I was preparing to meet my maker. The transfer from our local hospital to the more advanced hospital in Norfolk, Virginia, appeared to take an act of God or an act of Shirley.

The surgeons who admitted me for emergency surgery in Norfolk read a never before revealed disclosure on the transfer notes from the surgeon who took out the gallbladder and drained the cyst with the germ superhighway: "pancreas is gangrene". Nowhere else had that information appeared. Not in his surgical notes a month before. Not in my patient chart. Not in the notes of the other handful of specialists who flitted in and out of my hospital room. Not in the first discharge notes. Not in the follow-up office visit. Not in the re-admission's consulting notes with other doctors. No one else not talking to us in the hospital knew this, wrote down anywhere or said to our faces the word "gangrene". No one ever came to Shirley and I and said, "We're sorry Mr. and Mrs. Vaughan, but that routine gallbladder surgery we just did, well, we saw while we were in there that you lost your pancreas."

Years later, during the trial of the medical malpractice lawsuit, expert witnesses testified that the surgeon had violated the "standard of care" in a variety of unimaginably reckless ways: The surgery was not necessary, as the inflammation in the pancreas and the cyst were resolving. There had been no CAT scan taken immediately prior to the surgery to justify or nullify the need for the insertion of the drain tube into the pancreas, a month-old scan was used instead. If there had been any reason to operate on the pancreas, it should have been done by a qualified surgeon in a more qualified facility.

At the magnet hospital in Norfolk, a qualified surgeon ladled out what was left of my pancreas in an unscheduled emergency total pancreatectomy. We initially felt lucky to finally land in a hospital that had been ranked ten times in the *U.S. News and World Report's* "America's Best Hospitals" edition. Less than five percent of U.S. hospitals are named a Magnet Hospital by the American Nurses Credentialing Center, and Norfolk was also one of these. Magnet hospitals "have a strong culture of cooperation among nurses and physicians, which enhances patient safety and improves quality outcomes," says its Web site.

These sorts of code and medical speak on hospital Web sites were bits of information we missed back then because we didn't know to look for them. If a hospital mentions something like, they have a plan for patient safety or have been recognized as having a plan by an independent third party, this *should* mean something important to the *patient*. Something so important that your life could depend upon it. Is there any way an education in patient safety and advocacy could spare the two million people a year who contract hospital infections, or the 99,000 who die? You would like to think so. (This is why we have included a section at the end of this book for guidance, resources and support.)

I don't remember the ride home from Norfolk with my son and Shirley in our Monte Carlo. I don't think she does, either. The shock hadn't worn off for either of us. How was she supposed to take care of a man without a pancreas? Where were we supposed to find out how this was done when current medical literature said it couldn't be? The Norfolk hospital was state of the art, and their surgical team was amazing, but they sent us home with 30 minutes of training on an insulin pump and little guidance on what the coming weeks and months would hold. It wasn't their fault that they didn't know, even the U.S. Centers for Disease Control and Prevention, CDC, does not have statistics on total pancreatectomies or those surviving without a pancreas for any reason. Neither does the National Center for Health Statistics.

When I lost my pancreas, I became an instant brittle diabetic, without insulin to take food to my cells or enzymes to digest what food I would be allowed to eat. The new insulin pump was going to replace one job of my disintegrated pancreas: regulate my blood glucose levels. The stash of pills from the hospital pharmacy included medical grade enzymes to digest food, the other job of the pancreas. Only continuous human testing with a glucometer, another piece of equipment, would detect and help to prevent fatal insulin shock from blood glucose lows – a job the glucagon, also produced by my pancreas, used to do. The insulin pump had to be constantly monitored, cleaned, loaded, and because of my extensive abdominal surgical scarring, the pump's "ice pick" needle had to be mounted and plugged into my rear where I couldn't see it or get to it. This duty became one of the many new jobs for Shirley, who reminded me she swore being a nurse was one career she would never do.

As the shock wore off and we found ourselves trying to decipher computer equipment that would keep me alive, find doctors to give us clues and eliminate foods that wouldn't kill me, we were finding out the hard way what Gary Scheiner took time to reveal to diabetics in his book, *Think Like A Pancreas: A Practical*

Guide To Managing Diabetes with Insulin, [2] which was released the same summer I lost my pancreas: "In this age of assembly-line health care, dictated by third party managed care organizations, most physicians are limited in the amount of time they can spend with their patients. After taking vitals, reviewing histories and lab results, performing physical exams, ordering new lab work, and writing prescriptions, precious little time is available for your physician to sit down with you to teach you the finer points of living with diabetes and controlling your blood sugar levels."

This was Scheiner's advice to *traditional* diabetics, not surgically induced brittle diabetics: Predicting the stock market, the weather or the next five World Series winners could be "simpler" than managing your diabetes with insulin. Great. And this guy knows what he is talking about. Scheiner is a diabetic, a certified diabetes educator, insulin pump trainer, on the board of directors of the Diabetes Exercise and Sports Association and a volunteer for the American Diabetes Association.

I lost my pancreas to medical incompetence and error, and now I would be kept alive by medical ingenuity and Shirley's attention to detail, log keeping and cooking. We had nothing but time on our hands to think about things, like, how did this happen and how are we going to survive? All those car rides in the Monte Carlo with a broken radio and only our thoughts to share on things like survival, and how did they do it, now moved to the front of our minds instead of the back for getaway days. The hypothesizing was now a full-blown, ongoing real life, medical experiment. There would be no more getaways for a long time.

Some days, through the haze of little sleep and shattered nerves, we remembered the feel of sun on our faces and the wind in our hair, peering over wave tops toward a crumbling church tower on a forested riverbank. It was the metaphorical twin brothers of progress and efficiency who landed at Jamestown 400 years ago and dictated the terms of the takeover of the continent according to the principles of the revered industrial paradigm. As Shirley and I discovered, their rules are still in play with every aspect of American life, most certainly health care. Like human cogs injected into the machinery of modern medicine, Shirley and I began the grinding, long and difficult first year of navigating profound medical ignorance in the form of dismissive doctors, mastering the insulin pump, which can break and are occasionally recalled, monitoring insulin amounts – which Shirley regards as noxious and tries to keep as little as possible going into my body – preventing my sudden death from blood glucose drops and insulin shock, discovering a diet that worked and eventually, uncovering causes of an emerging mystery illness that wreaked havoc with our every effort to maintain my blood glucose levels and our sanity until we finally were forced to move from our home.

Every shred of our attention to detail and effort to chronicle our lack of progress through bone-tired exhaustion would be necessary on the coming roller coaster ride of skyrocketing and tanking blood glucose levels that lay ahead of us. The ride would prove too much for me that first winter without a pancreas, as my overloaded body gave up. I turned off my brain and the insulin pump, laid it on the kitchen counter and walked into the woods behind my home in search of lost peace — and death.

CHAPTER TWO:

Beyond Brittle: Taking Inventory,
Seeking Perspective

"He who has health, has hope. And he who has hope, has everything."

—Thomas Carlyle

Living without my pancreas meant my daily Herculean task was to master the components of surgically-induced diabetes and all of its fluctuating, life-threatening variables. As I found out, for all practical and technical purposes, calling my "condition" diabetes wasn't exactly correct. While true diabetics have pancreases with insufficient insulin to lower their blood glucose levels, they most likely will have insulin's opposite pancreas-produced hormone, glucagon, which prevents blood glucose from dropping too low. Glucagon also stimulates the release of insulin, so that glucose can be taken up and used by insulin-dependent tissues. So, glucagon and insulin are part of a feedback system that keeps blood glucose at precisely balanced levels.[1]

It is the blood glucose drops that can kill, which is why living without a pancreas is a more death-defying act that tackling traditional insulin-deficient only, Type 1 diabetes alone. Type 1 diabetics, who struggle to keep tight control of their blood glucose levels with strict diets, testing and insulin injections, are often referred to as "brittle" diabetes. Because of the lack of medical information on total pancreatectomies, TPs, there is no way to know how many patients are diabetic before going into their surgery, but this is where we all will end up, as I call us, "beyond brittle" diabetics. My challenge and that of any TP survivor was to find a way to scale the stratospheric learning curve of diabetes, including its insightful history as the oldest disease known to humankind, current medical science perspectives and pioneering, albeit profitable and sometimes questionable, tools for its necessary daily management.

In my self-studies in breakthrough moments of clarity, I found it curious that we, as in the human population of the planet, have experienced, documented and known about diabetes as a disease for thousands of years but are just now facing an epidemic of this disease, through both Type 1, a lack of pancreatic insulin, and Type 2, a modern diet-induced form of diabetes related to insulin resistance. Most any diabetes book or Web site you visit today fingers the blame for this epidemic to modern food systems born from the industrial ideals of progress and efficiency injected into a New World at the Jamestowne site, a mere 400 years ago. Medical science freely admits the relationship between industrially grown and processed food and diabetes is undeniably true — and well documented.

When the Sarah Constant (not Susan, as previously thought), the Godspeed and the Discovery sailed up an uncharted river and onto the sandy banks of the New World, doctors in the Old World were treating patients diagnosed with diabetes with "gelly of viper's flesh". This may sound, well, medieval, but dozens of variations of snake preparations – including snake wine and the maligned snake oil — were considered potent curatives for myriad illnesses for centuries. (Think of medicine's caduceus with the twin snakes wrapped around the staff.)

As the 1819 *American Edition of the British Encyclopedia* states, "The viper, though so much dreaded on account of its bite, has been very highly esteemed, both by the ancients and moderns, as a restorative and strengthening diet. The ancients used the flesh of this snake in leprous and other cases… In France and Italy, the broth, jelly, and flesh of vipers are in much esteem as a restorative medicine. In England we have to instance the well known circumstance of Sir Kenelm Digby, who caused his wife, Lady Venetia, to feed on capons fatted with vipers, to recover her from a consumption."[2]

I read the above passage about diabetics being treated with viper's jelly and then gratefully pat the small, computerized gadget hanging from my belt that Shirley attaches to my rear. On the other hand, further research revealed the insulin that was keeping me alive was derived from cow or pigs and then injected through recombinant DNA technology into an E. Coli bacterial cell – yes, the same bacteria transmitted through fecal-oral contaminations and responsible for regular national food recalls.

Insulin from animals – including sharks by the Japanese – was commonly used to treat diabetes in the early 20th century. In 1922, pharmaceutical giant Eli Lilly began commercial production of purified animal insulin. Fifty years later, pharmaceutical companies decided to inject the animal insulin into the E. Coli cells to create a genetically-engineered insulin that they would pass off as "human" insulin, which, of course, it is not. [3] And the jury is still out on whether the biosynthesized version of insulin is superior to its natural, animal alternative.

A 2005 study of comparing the "human" insulin to the animal version declared that, "A comparison of the effects of human and animal insulin as well as of the adverse reaction profile did not show clinically relevant differences. Many patient-oriented outcomes like health-related quality of life or diabetes complications and mortality were never investigated in high-quality, randomised clinical trials. The story of the introduction of human insulin might be repeated by contemporary launching campaigns to introduce pharmaceutical and technological innovations that are not backed up by sufficient proof of their advantages and safety." [4]

Translation: the porcine insulin DNA, which differs from human insulin DNA by one amino acid, was perfectly fine to use for diabetics, but pharmaceutical companies need patented products to push in the marketplace and so they created the engineered, patented product to peddle without a true need or rigorous testing to justify the so-called bio-synthetic "human" insulin.

Pharmaceutical companies stated this new engineered insulin was necessary because some patients' immune systems would recognize the bovine or porcine insulin as a foreign substance and produce antibodies against it, neutralizing its actions and resulting in inflammatory responses. However, studies show non-human insulin and genetically-engineered "human" insulin alike can cause allergic reactions in a tiny number of people and it is usually the preservatives used in the insulin, rather than the insulin molecule itself, responsible for the reaction.

Further complicating the ongoing argument over the superiority of natural vs. artificial insulin was a Wikipedia article stating, while biosynthetic "human" insulin has largely replaced animal insulin, the animal insulin is purer. "With the advent of high-pressure liquid chromatography (HPLC) equipment, the level of purification of animal-sourced insulins has reached as high as 99%, whereas the purity level of synthetic human insulins made via recombinant DNA has only attained a maximum purity level of 97%, which raises questions about the claim of synthetic insulin's purity relative to animal-sourced insulin varieties." [5]

Considering this new information, I paused while patting my pump and wondered, *what would viper's jelly on toast points taste like?*

How long has humankind known about diabetes? In 1552 BCE, Egyptian physician Hesy-Ra made the first known mention of diabetes – found on the Ebers Papyrus – and listed remedies to combat the "passing of too much urine". Nearly two thousand years later, Greek physician Aretaeus of Cappodocia coined the term "diabetes" from the Greek verb διαβαίνειν, or "diabaínein" meaning "to stride, walk, or stand with legs asunder"; hence, its derivative "diabētēs" meant "one that straddles." [6] A poor diabetic soul would be straddling often in the ancient world as the disease's main symptom was excessive urination. Aretaeus rendered the first complete medical description of diabetes as "the melting down of flesh and limbs into urine." Aretaeus did attempt to treat the disease but could not give a good prognosis; he commented that "life (with diabetes) is short, disgusting and painful."

Diabetes probably never disappeared from any human population, but it first appears in the English language as the Middle English word "diabete" in 1425. Sixty-eight years after the colonists on ships commissioned by the London Company founded Jamestowne Settlement, in 1675, Professor Thomas Willis of Oxford University described in his treatise *Pharmaceutice rationalis*, the "wonderfully sweet flavor" of urine in patients exhibiting symptoms of diabetes. And thus, a new diagnostic test for diabetes was born: urine tasting. Urine tasting as a method of monitoring blood sugars continued for over three centuries after Willis' death. [7]

It would be another century, 1776, in the same year the New World colonist declared their independence from the Old World, before English physician Matthew Dobson of Liverpool evaporated two quarts of urine from a patient with diabetes and conclusively established the presence of "saccharine materials" as a diagnosis of diabetes. But, perhaps the most glorious day in possibly all of medical history was in January 1922, when the Canadian surgeon Frederick Banting and his assistant Charles Best first successfully injected insulin into a dying child. After reversing a dog's diabetes, Banting and Best injected insulin into Leonard Thompson, a 14-year-old diabetic who lay dying at the Toronto General Hospital. The insulin was so impure at first that Thompson suffered a severe allergic reaction. A second purified dose was injected on January 23 with success.

During the early 20th century, children dying from diabetes were kept in large wards, often with 50 or more patients in a ward; most lay comatose as their grieving families awaited their inevitable death. As the story goes, after Thompson's recovery, Banting and Best went from bed to bed, injecting an entire ward with purified insulin. Before they had reached the last dying child, the first few were awakening from their comas to the joyous exclamations of their families.

For this, Banting and Best received the Nobel Prize in Physiology or Medicine in 1923; both shared their Prize money with others in the team who were not recognized. In an amazing gesture representing the noblest ideas of medicine, the scientists sold the patent for insulin was to the University of Toronto for one dollar and without attempts to control commercial production. Insulin production and therapy rapidly spread around the world, largely as a result of this humanitarian decision. Banting is annually honored by World Diabetes Day which is held on his birthday, November 14.

The pharmaceutical giant Eli Lilly produced large quantities of highly refined insulin from animals until the first patented and genetically-engineered, synthetic "human" insulin was produced in a laboratory in 1977 using E. coli. Eli Lilly sold the first commercially available biosynthetic human insulin under the brand name Humulin in 1982. The vast majority of insulin currently used worldwide is now biosynthetic recombinant "human" insulin or its analogs.

Once purified insulin was available, the challenge for diabetes became to know what their glucose levels were, and then to deliver the insulin via injections in amounts that would not lead to insulin shock or death from accidental overdose. Until the first portable glucose meter, created in 1969, diabetics were not able to regularly test themselves. The first glucometer was intended to help emergency room physicians distinguish between unconscious diabetics and unconscious drunks when the laboratories were closed at night.

While today, diabetics are certainly grateful to have an ability to manage their blood glucose levels at home, most do not realize that their meter readings can legally register up to 20 percent off the mark, leading to undetected lows or highs, and administration of too much insulin to counter the false readings. In an attempt to educate doctors, who were told the device was never meant to be used in a professional setting to replace laboratory testing, the FDA held a public hearing meeting on May 1, 2010 to consider recommendations to tighten the allowable error in glucometer readings to 10 percent. [8]

Despite testimonies from doctors citing the glucometers regular use in a variety of hospital treatment protocols in probably "billions of times each year", a manufacturer representative present at the 2010 hearing said the over-the-counter glucometers "was never intended for patients on tight glycemic control in the hospital setting." An FDA representative said the agency receives 12,000 adverse-event reports each year involving glucose meters. More than 12,000 serious adverse events associated with glucose meters were reported during 2004–08, and FDA has investigated 100 deaths related to the devices since 1992.

The findings of the FDA hearing were a "consensus" for "the need for better analytical and clinical performance of glucose meters, better labeling and identification of substances that interfere with meter performance, and better glucose targets for hospitalized patients".

Once the issue of self-testing was solved, sort of, by portable, calculator-sized glucometers, the challenge of administering properly timed and adequate amounts of insulin was overcome with the first insulin pump, designed in the '70s to mimic the body's normal release of insulin. The pump dispenses a continuous insulin dosage through a plastic tube, using a small needle that is inserted into the skin. The first pumps were large and bulky and had to be carried in a backpack. The pump I use now is lightweight enough to hang from my belt buckle. [8]

Other devices that companies are coming up with to cash in on the current epidemic of diabetes have included a glucometer that would work as a wrist watch. But it could fail when the skin would become sweaty and hot, according to a March 2001 US Food and Drug Administration report.[9] Also in development is a gadget to integrate the glucose meter and a cell phone. [10]

One savvy online blogger evaluated these needle-free devices and decided they belonged in the same class as Bigfoot than reality for a reason – their success would eliminate a billion dollar source of profit for pharmaceutical companies: testing strips. "I have looked forward to the GlucoWatch for years. But I have recently decided to place this hourly automatic blood testing watch in a class with the Bigfoot, the abominable snowman and Goldilocks. Yeah, it's a myth.

"When I was first diagnosed with diabetes, more than 10 years ago, the diabetic nurse told me that there were new inventions that would make having diabetes easier. I was fascinated by the GlucoWatch and similar devices. This device promised to continuously monitor your blood sugar, it could give you a graph of your entire day's sugar readouts, it could sound an alarm when your blood sugar went out of range when you were sleeping. It was in testing for years…" writes the blogger. "Now we are told that diabetics will be able to implant meters that send data to their watches, or their cell phones. These 'glucophones' are not covered by insurance, require surgery for an implant, and yep you guessed it, are still in testing.

"It's enough to make me think there is a conspiracy afoot. Maybe the drug companies don't want to give up their dollar a test strip fortune. Or maybe a device that could measure your sugar continuously is too much to ask for."[11]

This blogger is right. Every time a diabetic wants to know what their blood glucose levels are before accidently under or overdosing with the wonder drug insulin, they will need to fork over one dollar, the same price the patent for insulin was sold to the University of Toronto by its Noble Prize-winning inventor. The pharmaceutical companies will generously give you a free glucose meter these days, because they know their real cash cow and the money pit for diabetics is the regular testing required to stay alive. For the average Type 1 diabetic who uses 10 to 12 strips a day, that adds up to $4,000 a year. The cost is even higher for a "beyond brittle" diabetic who may test continuously that first year after a total pancreatectomy.

According to industry consultants, the actual cost of manufacturing a test strip is only about eight to 12 cents and the vendors make about a 60-80% profit on each box, or possibly even higher. The US market for diabetic patient monitoring systems is expected to reach $9.1 billion by 2010.[12] Reports of diabetics foregoing testing due to the expense of strips and a thriving black market for questionable quality testing strips are regularly featured in diabetes magazines. The prohibitive expense of testing strips for some means a greater risk of diabetes complications, and therefore, greater health care expenses for all of us, not to mention early death for diabetics.

If diabetes is left untreated and blood glucose levels consistently become too high, red blood cells harden into crusty sugar-coated crystals that tear small capillaries in the extremities of the body. This is why diabetics are at risk for blindness, amputations, comas and kidney failure. This sort of damage, called neuropathy, even though it can lead to death, usually takes place over a long period of time. On the opposite end, when a diabetic's blood glucose levels become too low, they can have an insulin reaction, meaning there is too much insulin and not enough sugar in the blood so the cells begin to die. A severe drop in blood glucose levels could lead to insulin shock, a quick death for a diabetic. [13]

With the growing global epidemic of diabetes accelerating, it doesn't take a genius to notice the potential for profit is also endless. According to the American Diabetes Association, ADA, one in twenty Americans should plan their futures around managing diabetes and supporting the pharmaceutical industry with their health insurance premiums. Currently, diabetes was the seventh leading cause of death listed on U.S. death certificates in 2006. The International Diabetes Federation shows the disease affects 246 million people worldwide. [14]

How does an average person begin to comprehend the human instinct driving those noble physicians administering those first doses of life-saving insulin to dying diabetic children and then giving away their patent for the good of humanity to the reptilian instinct of the pharmaceutical industry to profit obscenely from the suffering of their fellow human beings? Once again, the question of "who serves whom" and how to inject a heart into the machinery of modern industrial-modeled medicine begs to be answered.

Even though the history of diabetes was long and glorious, the history of living without a pancreas was not. The guidance Shirley and I needed to help us find our way through the coming months of transitioning me to living without this vital organ did not exist, and there was a reason for this, one that we would not discover until almost six years after my emergency TP.

Total pancreatectomies, TPs, had not found favor in the past with the medical establishment because of its high morbidity rate – meaning you would die without your pancreas. However, a study dated May 20, 2010 and posted on PubMed, the website of the US National Library of Medicine, examined 65 TPs between 1996 and 2008. Apparently, 65 TPs in twelve years are not enough to create a representative, traceable sample for the CDC or NCHS.

The study, conducted by the University of Verona, Italy, explained, "Total pancreatectomy (TP) has been performed rarely in the past because of its high morbidity and mortality. Because outcomes of pancreatic surgery as well as management of pancreatic insufficiency have improved markedly, enthusiasm for TP has increased." The study concluded that, "TP can be performed safely with no mortality and acceptable morbidity. Postoperative pancreatic insufficiency can be managed safely... TP is an effective operation in selected patients." [15]

According to our experience, "selected" patients must be the key term here and mean patients who have someone to care for them 24/7, or who can afford around the clock nursing care necessary for the first few months to a year. We truly don't know how else this is done – living without a pancreas – unless you have constant human care.

One other German study from 2008 asked as its title, "Is there still a role for Total Pancreatectomy." The study's abstract states, "TP was abandoned for decades because of high peri- and postoperative morbidity and mortality. Because selected pancreatic diseases are best treated by TP, and pancreatic surgery and postoperative management of exocrine and endocrine insufficiency have significantly improved, the hesitance to perform a TP is disappearing." [16]

We did not find other current American studies or universities that expand on the possibilities of TPs becoming a mainstream medical operation. Curious, we did poll American universities and hospitals, both by phone and email through their media departments, to ask for help in compiling individual hospital statistics since the national centers did not track or maintain such rare statistics on TPs. Most university hospitals' media officers could not offer us information, though many were nice and wished us well on our search. The Johns Hopkins media officer pointed us to their message board where we posted a request for help, and found it through a small group of TP survivors who supported one another and shared their experiences through a Yahoogroup discussion board. Their shared stories echoed our own frustration at blindly navigating the first few years post-TP (and are shared at the end of this book).

The American Pancreatic Association said they were a professional membership group, run by volunteers, and they did not keep statistics of any kind. They did say, "it would depend upon who you spoke to find out if pancreatectomies are recommended or not." [17].

Understanding how slowly medical science can move at times, and then, when it does, how its profit-driven industrial paradigm determines what information and products are eventually marketed to the public, it is a quick commonsense leap to wonder: If medical science is "less hesitant" to perform TPS, and therefore, moving toward recommending total pancreatectomies as a preventive surgery for cancer or curative surgery for pancreatitis sufferers, how much longer will it be true that TP survivors are destined to become living medical experiments, participating in this barely acknowledged procedures' unpredictable, "beyond brittle" diabetic aftermath?

Taking inventory of the high tech, pricey gadgets pharmaceutical companies are able to come up with to help diabetics manage their disease, from my vantage point, there is a huge gap in all of this equipment, "something" that will be necessary for beyond brittle TP survivors: nowhere is there listed the one necessary *human being* that will stay by your side, compensate for the variety of mechanical failures possible, take your blood glucose readings when you are on the verge of insulin shock, cook you meals until you are mobile, and in all, help you survive that first year post-TP surgery.

I have no doubt that, had it not been for my wife's constant care that first year, I would not be here to tell this tale. All the self-education and hindsight of our situation would come years later, after my suicide attempt, after we discovered how on our own we were, after the medical malpractice suit, after the mystery illness was solved and finally, after our return to our roots, with all of its common sense healing possibilities.

CHAPTER THREE:

I Become a Living Medical Experiment and Shirley Becomes A Lot of Things

]"It's supposed to be a secret, but I'll tell you anyway. We doctors do nothing.

We only help, And encourage the doctor within."

—Albert Schweitzer, M.D.

So, I left the Norfolk hospital in September 2004 without my pancreas and as an instant, beyond brittle diabetic. At a skeletal 128 pounds at 5' 10", with a stomach that had not processed food for months, and arms and legs that had stiffened with lack of function in a hospital bed, my son and Shirley drove a near corpse to our home two hours away where I would begin my life as a living medical experiment and Shirley would begin her life as a nurse, researcher, dietician, data cruncher, and night guard. The doctor who discharged me from Norfolk predicted that, without a pancreas, I would never put on weight again. I told him to just let me out of there and get home to my wife's cooking and we'd see about that.

An insulin pump now took on the role of providing my body with biosynthetic "human" insulin to transport nutrients into my cells. Like every other technological gadget, insulin pumps have potentials for life-threatening glitches and recalls are not unheard of – neither are deaths from a failed pump. In 2004, Medtronic recalled over 160,000 insulin pumps due to a defective tube. That episode led to at least 200 diabetic patients being injured and/or hospitalized, and at least one fatality. In 2009, the same company recalled an estimated three million of the infusion sets that come with the pump. Over or under delivery of insulin from an insulin pump could have catastrophic consequences for diabetes patients.[1] (Instead of trading in the defective pump for a new one, one savvy product liability law firm warned diabetics who were told to "turn in" their pumps, not to do so.[2])

And then there are the US Food and Drug Administration's warnings for testing strips that were giving diabetics "falsely elevated blood glucose results" because they could not "distinguish between glucose and other sugars... including maltose, xylose, and galactose." The 2009 FDA warning pointed out that, "These sugars can falsely elevate glucose results, which may mask significant hypoglycemia or prompt excessive insulin administration, leading to serious injury or death."[3]

As Shirley and I were getting ready to discover, a common sense approach that machinery like glucometers, testing strips and pumps can fail, encouraged us to be vigilant and WRITE EVERYTHING DOWN. Eventually, either the machine or the person could break down and a written record of a patient's diabetes management will be the real life-saving device, as it became for us.

Our 30 minute insulin pump orientation before leaving the hospital, and while we were still in shock, helped to point us in the right direction. The home nurse that Medicare paid to stop by and check my vitals and feed me through a stomach tube, helped to ease our terror over being left completely on our own the first few weeks, but her commission ran out and it was just Shirley and I in our home, studying the pump and glucometer for clues on how things were going with my body's adjustment to living without my pancreas.

"I used to think you had a cute butt," Shirley cracked often, while attaching the unit to my rear for the umpteenth time. "But now that I have to look at it all the time, I'm not so sure!"

My fingers became scabbed over with constant pricking with an automatic lancet device, a pointed piece of surgical steel encased in plastic used to draw the drop of blood I inserted on the pricey, hopefully not on the recall list, test strips which were then inserted into the glucometer whose test results were legally allowed to be 20 percent off. A diabetic really has only six fingers to work with if you leave out the too sensitive thumbs and two too small pinkies. I began to rotate which fingers were the least scabbed over and ended up losing the use of two all together for testing. Only four were left to serve up that crucial drop of blood that would tell us how our home-based medical experiment with iffy equipment was going.

At least a thousand times, while wincing and squeezing a drop of my own blood from a purple finger, I promised myself if I ever became a millionaire I would hire one of those genius MIT graduate students to find out how much surface area is really available on a fingertip for pricking with a not-so-needlelike lancet for the precious drop of blood that was necessary to know if I am going to live or die.

The experimental testing formula would need to go something like this: Surface area of finger multiplied by still usable fingertips divided by the lancet sized hole and its surrounding sore area equals how many sore holes you can make total. Once you know how many times you can punch a hole in the most nerve-ending-riddled and sensitive parts of your body (don't forget the squeezing out the blood drop part if the hole isn't big enough) you could then divide by the minutes in the day and know how often you could take your own blood without having to hit the same sore spots over and over again. But really, we diabetics already know the answer to this riddle: you don't miss the sore spots because they don't heal instantly. We read various institutions' recommendations for avoiding sore fingertips and tried not to smirk at their uselessness when drawing so much blood so often. The common advice to prick the sides of your fingers and not the tips was undone by the countering confessions that the sides of your fingers are not as blood rich as the padded sensitive parts. What really happens is the fingertips scab over and toughen-up and you reset the lancet's depth to shoot the surgical steel point deeper on its next jab into the doomed digit.

It's true that some meters offer alternate site testing, which allows testing on areas other than the fingertips. However, alternate site testing is not as accurate as finger pricks and you still have to repeat the test on a fingertip if it is too high or low. This can be a real problem if a person is already on the low side. A false higher reading may prompt a correction bolus dose of insulin when in fact, the person is already, or heading into, a state of low blood sugar. So sticking with the fingertips was a no-brainer for me.

In addition to logging our lives and poking the pump into my rear, another skill honed by Shirley that saved me many nights was her mother's ability - unappreciated by our children - to sit straight up in bed fully awake at the slightest sound, especially a floor board creaking. "I know what every board in every room in this house sounds like Clyde, so don't bother trying to let me off the hook to sleep," she scolded me when I was finally able to get out of bed and wait on myself. It was true. If I was in the kitchen going for a snack to counter a blood glucose drop, the board in front of the pantry would betray me in my half asleep daze every time.

Then there were the times, too many to remember, that I didn't wake up. This was the norm in the beginning: taking my blood sugar readings every two hours around the clock, all through the night. Shirley said when I wouldn't wake up she would shake me until I gave her that deer in the headlights look and she would feel better before pricking one of my sore, overworked four digits and then either feeding me, waiting to test again, or going back to bed for another two hours.

On the nights that we gave up on sleep, we learned things about our neighbors that we didn't know before. Some of this new information was entertaining and some of it downright scary. Some of the smoke rolling out of one home's windows turned out to not be a kitchen fire. One of the teenagers appeared to have a drive-thru business of sorts running out of his bedroom window. And one woman, down at the end of the street, saw so many cars coming and going in one night we blushed at the thoughts we had, until we saw the sheriff's deputy drive up early in the morning, apparently not on business. And then we thought we best just pull down our own blinds and speculations. We do live in a small town, but the drama is never small.

At some point, we had the presence of mind and strength to begin to log *everything*: the time we checked my blood glucose readings, to insulin doses to exact quantities of food and how they affected the glucometer readings. We also added a second glucometer to our regime of testing to double check a string of unusual or suspicious test results. All of these bits of information tied together became a life raft for us on the rolling ocean swells of super high blood sugar readings, drops that knocked me out and overshoots with Coke that would send me back up again.

By October, the swings from the highs and lows had taken its toll on both of us. My brain and body were finished. They just wanted to switch off and rest a while. What a far away and crazy notion our dream of peace was during those days. But I think this is what I wanted, just peace. Thinking clearly isn't possible with diabetics with poor blood glucose control, much less out-of-control blood glucose levels. Thinking clearly became impossible for me two months after I lost my pancreas.

And then, I guess I had just had it. Through a half-crazed haze I must have navigated the squeaky boards one night to make sure Shirley didn't wake up. The insulin pump needle jammed in my rump that hurt constantly from having to learn to sit on it came out with one tug as I tossed the whole contraption onto the kitchen counter and walked out the back door. Whatever kind of existence this was, it was torture and I was done with it. I could die without the pump delivering the insulin to my body, but I didn't care.

Within an hour, Shirley found the insulin pump on the counter and started calling our children. Two came right away and drove through our neighborhood in the rain and dark looking for their Dad. When they didn't find me, they called the sheriff and got help searching for me in the woods. I don't remember much after this, as my body was following my brain in shutting down.

From what my children and Shirley told me later, the sheriff found me when his patrol car lights shined through the woods at the end of our neighborhood. I was dazed, but conscious, even standing up and shivering in the rain. Because the sheriff had been called, my attempted suicide was now a legal issue and the police and state were charged with protecting my life, even from myself.   An emergency squad transported me to a hospital for stabilization, where my family and I waited and waited for word to come back of where I was going to go next.

Who was going to take me in and oversee my mental recovery from the trauma of losing my pancreas and becoming a surgically-induced diabetic? And this is when we found out just how on our own we were: no one wanted me. No hospital in the Commonwealth of Virginia wanted to be responsible for keeping alive a depressed man without a pancreas. They had no idea how to do this and weren't going to put themselves in that position. The same ambulance, ordered by the sheriff whose sworn legal duty was to protect me from myself and delivery me to the safety of medical professionals who had taken similar oaths, took me back home later the same night, hours after I decided I rather die than live like a medical experiment anymore.

Back home, my family quietly helped me to bed, where the rounds and rounds of testing my glucose every two hours and adjusting the reattached pump and guessing which foods I could tolerate would begin all over again as if my giving up and walking into the woods had never happened.

Surrender came. But not defeat. Not as long as my shoeless angel hovered over my body, moonlight or daylight, and did not give up. Shirley did not give up. Her logs and calendars and cooking and love did not fail us during this time. Or her humor.

"Oh great, get ready, here comes Dr. Frankenstein," she whispered to me in the endocrinologist's examination room after a somber Christmas. And sure enough, there was the oldest physician in the world, practiced for more than 50 years, bent over, holding onto the wall, and creeping toward us as we waited in the chilly room.

The drive to an endocrinologist's office – a doctor who manages diabetic patients - was an hour one way to Chesapeake, Virginia. When we finally did arrive to the month's-in-advance booked appointment, we found out the physician we were there to see had left town, but provided his patients with a temporary replacement.

I think it hurt to laugh, but Shirley's wicked gleam and dead on mimicry of the ancient doctor behind his back did me in. "Wonder if he's got some viper jelly left over from his glory days for me?" I whispered to Shirley. We both did our best to contain the welcome giggle attack.

The physician didn't say hello, or want to look at Shirley's meticulous logs, which got her ire up even more. I scooted down the exam table a little ways to make room for any impending foot stomping dances. "You'll need to see the pump specialist," was his dictate before skulking away with no eye contact, and no foot dancing… lucky fellow.

The pump specialist turned out to be a young lady who worked in the shared office with the endocrinologist's patients.

"We were told we need to see you today," said Shirley to the young woman at the reception desk.

"No, you'll have to make an appointment to see me," she replied.

"We made an appointment to be here months ago," corrected Shirley.

"You have to make a different appointment to see me," she informed.

"We have to drive an hour each way for these appointments. Can't you see us today since we are here?" asked Shirley, making a point of looking around at the lack of busyness the pump specialist seemed engaged in at the time.

"No, you'll have to make an appointment," said the specialist, unbending and unknowingly testing Shirley's tapping toes. I backed toward the door, but my evasive maneuvering was unnecessary as our watch told us it was time to take another blood glucose reading before hopping into the car and heading home. Shirley took the pump specialist's business card.

We would like to say we never went back. But endocrinologists and their minions of assistants are rare and hard to come by in our neck of the woods. Shirley says they know it, which is why they are fine with tending to their rules instead of their patients. The specialist recalibrated the pump and retrained Shirley to stick it to me with the pump's ice pick on our return, and properly booked, visit.

The weariness of our first winter seemed to lessen a little as the weather warmed. Spring came, and I was able to sit outside in the swings near the boxwood maze for short spells. The earth was starting to smell of promises and the nights still cool when I spotted a little miracle surrounded by pine needles in a bed in the front yard. A rare and wild orchid, a pink lady slipper, had pushed up between two hedges against the warm brick wall of the house.

I called for Shirley to come and look at this small flower. She knew as well as I did this endangered forest flower did not grow outside its home. It rarely grew anywhere anymore, as it had been discovered by New World settlers and their progeny who overharvested the species in the past centuries for its medicinal roots... used for depression.

We looked up and down our asphalt street and toward our neighbors' homes, whose secrets we now knew. Where could it have come from? How did it get here, and when? There are professionals trying to grow these orchids in captivity and failing, and here one shows up in our front yard. Shirley and I marveled together over its exotic venous, bulbous form. We both got down on our knees to get a good look at it and make sure we were really seeing the rare flower. Despite being harvested to the point of extinction, to being a forest flower and nearly impossible to grow, it found a way to live. And right here. But how? Maybe it blew up the road and out of the woods at the end of our street. The same woods I took a death wish walk in the previous fall.

"God didn't say we would get a perfect life," said Shirley, holding my hand and sharing her favorite prayerful chant. "But he did say He would never leave us." We suddenly realized we had never been abandoned. Not once. We would need this reminder again and again in the coming years as we faced a battering medical malpractice suit and a forced relocation from our beloved family home to ease the symptoms of a devastating mystery illness, which wasn't a mystery for long.

CHAPTER FOUR:

Why We Sued the Doctor and Why We Lost the Case

"I find medicine is the best of all trades because whether you do any good or not you still get your money."

– Moliere, *A Physician in Spite of Himself*, 1664

By the time Shirley and I navigated through the first year, we were beginning to realize the truth. The surgeon hadn't killed me with his incompetence or the hospital with its contagions, or the medical community in general with their lack of knowledge to guide us. I was going to live. We didn't know for how long, but the mounting costs for my care were taking a toll on both of us financially, physically and emotionally.

We decided to visit an attorney to see what our options were. Shirley packed up our travel kit and made sure the latches were locked in case we were pulled over by a police officer who, in Virginia, could legally charge us with transporting drug paraphernalia with the load of medical supplies it carried if it were not locked.

The attorney we hired filed our lawsuit against the surgeon in 2006, almost at the deadline for filing a medical malpractice case. Not being able to participate much in the trial preparation, we laid low and allowed our attorneys to do their jobs over the next two years. The attorney, Shirley and I felt the medical malpractice case was clear cut given the fact that I no longer had a pancreas. Personally, my biggest concern was the lawyers' abilities — on both sides — to put together an unbiased jury. As it turned out, the narrow definition of what constitutes a "celebrity" prevented us from holding the trial in a different, larger town. That was a joke, in case you missed it.

Sure, I'm not "famous" according to *People* magazine or the *National Enquirer*, but in the small town where I had lived my entire life, digging up and compiling a jury of my peers who weren't related to me, or someone I knew, or whose family member might have a grudge against my son, a supervisor at the local paper mill for two decades, or someone whose family cow had a beef with my family's cow sometime during the last century, was going to be a challenge, in my opinion.

Genealogy and family heritage is taken very seriously in Southampton County, originally called Warrasquoyocke and one of eight shires making up the original Colony of Virginia. It is only speculation that the 600 square-mile area sharing a border with North Carolina was renamed after an English lord. Founded as an official county in 1749, with an official court building in 1752, in 2009 the Southampton courthouse became the first in American history to have all its records – from 1749 onward – digitized, on-line accessible, and indexed by every man, woman and child as well as land sites.

The county is rightfully proud of its agricultural history, but one story in its past is a dark blot that civic-minded residents actively address and overcome with education and preservation efforts. In 1831, the county was the scene of the infamous Nat

Turner's Rebellion, also known as the Southampton Insurrection, the bloodiest slave rebellion in American history.

Nat Turner, an enslaved African-American minister was called a "prophet" by whites and blacks during his lifetime. As a child, it was acknowledged that he possessed clairvoyant abilities and said he spoke to God. As an adult, Turner felt God called him to lead his people from bondage by planning and carrying out the slave uprising in August 1831 that killed 60 white people – mostly children — and led to the retaliatory deaths of between 100 to 200 enslaved African-Americans. The victims of the uprising – including an infant - were mostly decapitated, hacked or stabbed to death. The murders included my great-great-great grandfather's niece, Rebecca Vaughan. The tavern that stood down the street from the courthouse was run by Rebecca and her family. Her house now stands in the Southampton County Heritage Village and Agriculture/Forestry Museum, two blocks from my house. The museum's sign in front of the house states the home's historic significance: it is the site of the last murders of the Southampton Insurrection, as the town militia stopped the slaughters before the mob crossed over the Flower Bridge and into Jerusalem, the original name of our township. What the sign doesn't say is blood stains from the murders are still visible on the wood floor planks in the upstairs of the house, according to local and family rumor. A $420,000 federal grant is currently restoring the home which will house an electronic driving tour of the Insurrection route through the county.[1]

Turner was eventually captured and tried in Jerusalem, and he and 20 to 50 of his followers were hanged, depending upon which account you read. Turner himself was hanged, decapitated, dissected and skinned on November 11, 1831. His own account of the events of his life were transcribed before his execution and preserved in *The Confession of Nat Turner*, although the accuracy of the confession is questioned by some. [2] The insurrection and its far-reaching aftermath are considered to be a critical spark in the powder keg of racial tensions and the acknowledgement of the abomination of slavery – the engine of those ideas of progress and efficiency that landed at Jamestowne — that exploded into the Civil War, and eventually ended in slavery's abolishment.

Just because the stories of Virginia's past are everywhere and a part of our daily lives, they are not taken for granted or ignored. They still whisper lessons to us relevant to our "modern" lives if we take the time to listen.

Our medical malpractice lawsuit against the surgeon who turned me into a living medical experiment and Shirley into a full-time nurse maid was heard by a "jury of my peers" and likely several times removed kin, and held in the 1834 courthouse built three years after the insurrection and on the site of the original 1752 courthouse. There are no points I am trying to make here. This is just what happened. The courthouse is three blocks in the other direction of our house. I wasn't kidding when I said we live in a small town.

By the time the lawsuit got underway, in late 2008 and four years after I lost my pancreas, Shirley and I had cracked the code on much of the diet and dosing needed to keep my blood glucose stable. We had also solved the mystery of my ongoing flu-like illness that would hit me every few weeks and leave me in bed or on the couch for days at a time. The smoke surrounding our neighborhood on fall and winter mornings was so toxic from household trash chemicals being released into the air from my neighbor's wood burning stove, my insulin was made ineffective, my body's inflammation and glucose readings soared and there was nothing to do but move out of our beloved family home. Our one street town did not sport apartment complexes, so, during the trial period, we were forced to live in a small apartment in the big, neighboring city of Franklin during the winters. Getting through the trial... well, it was a trial. But clarity over what had happened to my pancreas did emerge. Clarity emerged, right alongside craziness.

During the four days of hearings, we sat in the courtroom and listened to the surgeon with the impaired memory, who retired from practice before the trial began, crow like a rooster on the stand that "he knew my pancreas was gone the minute he opened me up!" I heard him in the months following in nightmares when I sat up in bed sweating from severe blood glucose drops and Shirley would rush in and hover over me, tipping Coke into my mouth and checking the readings until we could get the blood sugar level back up, and then sometimes, back down again.

As I warned you, I'm not going to bother to try to tell you what happened or who said what about what in this trial. I have tried to summarize the events, read my own words, and didn't believe them myself. So, instead of a second hand account, I am going to let you read the transcript for yourself, as I have done many times trying to discover the truth.

The following courtroom scene took place on November 13, 2008. The attorney asking the questions below is my attorney. He is questioning the surgeon who took out my gallbladder and then took it upon himself to install a tube to drain the pancreatic pseudocyst that had not been scanned or x-rayed during the month before the gallbladder surgery. This is the same surgeon who later said the hospital contagion didn't crawl up the drain tube he installed and infect my pancreas, because my pancreas was already "dry, black, dead" gangrenous tissue, and he just "FORGOT" to write this in any of his notes, tell any other doctors or inform his patient that he had just lost a major organ.

Attorney: And you decided at that time that no debridement, that is, you weren't going to remove the black, gangrenous, dead, pancreatic tissue, because that should be done only at a university hospital?

Surgeon: Correct.

Attorney: And it would require taking out the whole pancreas and the whole pancreas was necrotic, correct?

Surgeon: What I see. Yes, sir.

Attorney: And you didn't do it because that should be done only at a university hospital where they are better equipped to handle it?

Surgeon: Several reasons why I didn't do it. And that it – you just mentioned one.

Attorney: The reason why you didn't do it was because there was no infection?

Surgeon: The reason I didn't do it is I don't – I don't feel comfortable taking out or operating on the body and tail or taking out the whole pancreas. Two, there is no urgency in doing that operation at that time. The pancreas – I am not talking about the cyst – the body and tail of the pancreas is charcoaled, paper like and dry. There is no infection, active infection.

Attorney: There was – and that was another reason why you felt it was not necessary to send him to have his pancreas removed because there was no infection?

Surgeon: No.

Attorney: All right. It was not wet. It was like dry, gangrene, correct?

Surgeon: Correct. It is dry, gangrene.

Attorney: So there was no acute infection, no reason to have that pancreas taken out at that time?

Surgeon: Correct.

Attorney: Okay. And the liquid that – but even though his pancreas was dried, black and dead, you felt you should go ahead and drain the cyst on the pancreas?

Surgeon: The cyst is separated from the body and the tail of the pancreas. It is not – it is not the same – we are not talking about the same area. We divide the pancreas in three sections, the head, the body and the tail. And I work only in the head or the cyst that was situated in the head of the pancreas. I didn't touch the body and tail.

Attorney: So it is your testimony, Dr. Capati, that the body and tail of the pancreas was dry, charcoal, black and dead but the head was alive?

Surgeon: I didn't say that the head was alive.

Attorney: All right. But you're –

Surgeon: The head is occupied by a cyst.

Attorney: The head is occupied by a cyst but you decided to drain the cyst on a dead pancreas, is that what you are telling the jury?

Surgeon: I decided to drain the cyst. Correct.

Attorney: On a dead pancreas?

Surgeon: Yes, lying beside a dead pancreas.

Attorney: Okay. Doctor, is this – I am handing you a two-page document, and I am asking you: Is that your operative note from that day?

Surgeon: Yeah. Yeah.

Attorney: Would you like to refer to that or do you want to use your own?

Surgeon: I want to use my own. It is the same.

Attorney: Are you ready, sir?

Surgeon: Yes, sir.

Attorney: Now, Doctor, I am going to direct your attention to about right here. The top. See if you agree with me. About the top third of your note talks about the gallbladder?

Surgeon: Is that right?

Attorney: And I see on your page you have marked at the beginning the word "initially"?

Surgeon: That is right. That is where we start.

Attorney: That starts the part of your note that deals with the pancreas, correct?

Surgeon: Yes, sir.

Attorney: Go ahead and read that note to the jury, Doctor.

Here, the surgeon reads to the jury his complex surgical notes involving how he decided and did drain the baseball-sized cyst.

Attorney: So, Doctor, you would agree with me, wouldn't you, sir, that your operative note mentions nothing about the entire pancreas being dry, gangrenous, dead or black?

Surgeon: Yes, sir. I agree. I forgot that. I forgot that.

Attorney: You forgot to put that in your notes?

Surgeon: In my operative note. I forgot to dictate it.

Attorney: You forgot that?

Surgeon: Yes, sir.

Attorney: And did you also forget to put in there that you called Dr. Ketoff because of this dry, black condition of the pancreas? Did you forget to put that in there, too?

Surgeon: No. No.

Attorney: It doesn't say you called him for that, does it?

Surgeon: No. When I – after I made the opening in the capsule, since this case is unusual, and I felt that having another surgeon look at the case before I finished it or complete what I had in mind, to have him take a look – take a look at the operative findings and just see what he thinks about it.

Attorney: But the only thing you put in your note was that you and he discussed an internal versus an external drain. That is all that you said in your note that you and he talked about.

Surgeon: Read it. Yeah. That is true. But that doesn't mean that is the only thing we talk about. It was out there the whole operation at that time.

Attorney: That was the only thing you thought noteworthy to put in your note or did you simply just forget?

Surgeon: No. That I thought that was noteworthy to note.

Attorney: Maybe I haven't asked this question well. It wasn't noteworthy to put in your note that you and Dr. Ketoff talked about the dry, gangrene, dead pancreas?

Surgeon: He can see it. I can see it. I don't see the point in talking about it. I don't know. This is four years ago. I don't know exactly what we discussed. Couldn't remember that far.

Attorney: You dictated this note when? That day?

Surgeon: This one is dictated same day. Yeah.

Attorney: And the only thing you put in there that you and he discussed was an external versus internal drain?

Surgeon: This is the note that is written there because I thought that is the most important for whatever we discussed that day.

Attorney: And it wasn't important to put that the – his pancreas was dead because you weren't dealing with the pancreas?

Surgeon: I didn't say that. I just forgot it.

Attorney: You forgot that?

Surgeon: Yes, sir.

Attorney: Doctor, let me – do you have your discharge note?

Surgeon: Yes.

Attorney: Let me direct you to that, if you would, please, sir. Do you have it?

Surgeon: Yes, sir. I do.

Attorney: This is – this is your discharge summary dictated on September 4th, when Mr. Vaughan came out of the hospital after you did the cholecystectomy; correct?

Surgeon: Yes, sir.

Attorney: And in that you talk about what the discharge diagnosis is, you list what the operation was, you give a history, examination, hospital course. It is a summary of everything that happened?

Surgeon: Yes, sir.

Attorney: Correct?

Surgeon: Yes, sir. You are correct.

Attorney: Okay. In your discharge diagnosis, you put cholecystitis with cholelithiasis?

Surgeon: Yes, sir.

Attorney: History of pancreatitis?

Surgeon: Yes, sir.

Attorney: Pancreatic head pseudocyst?

Surgeon: Yes, sir.

Attorney: That is your final discharge diagnosis?

Surgeon: Correct.

Attorney: You didn't diagnose a dead, gangrenous, dry pancreas?

Surgeon: I didn't – I did not write it.

Attorney: Did you forget to write it there, too, Doctor?

Surgeon: Yes, sir.

The surgeon goes on to tell the court that he did not tell me what he found and his notes do not reflect that he told me my pancreas was dead. In fact, *he sent me home.* In our version of events, based on reality, I went home with a drainage tube exiting my body to recover from gallbladder surgery and having a cyst drained. Within a week, I lost ten pounds, began vomiting violently and having knee-buckling abdominal pain. I was readmitted to the hospital I had just left. The surgeon was called in for a "consult" by the other doctors, so they could benefit from his knowledge of my case. He once again "forgets" to tell these doctors that the man they are watching vomit violently lost his pancreas to gangrene a few weeks ago. This is a continuation of the same interview in the same day by my attorney.

Attorney: And you wrote a consultation note, didn't you, sir?

Surgeon: Yes, sir.

Attorney: Do you have that in front of you, dictated 9/9/04?

Surgeon: Yes, sir.

Attorney: The reason for the consultation was vomiting, weight loss and abdominal pain?

Surgeon: Yes, sir.

Attorney: And you have the history of the illness. And you and I am reading at Number 3, open cholecystectomy and draining of the pancreatic head cyst three weeks ago. At that time, he had a lot of necrosis in the head of the pancreas. Most appropriate treatment for drainage at the time was placing a Number 34 mushroom catheter through the mesentery on the underside of the transverse colon. That is what you wrote, isn't it, Doctor?

Surgeon: Yes, sir.

Attorney: Again, you didn't say anything on that admit consult about the history of the rest of the pancreas being dry, black or gangrene or charcoal, like paper or dead?

Surgeon: No. I didn't – I didn't write in there that the rest of the pancreas is dry, black and paper, charcoal.

Attorney: Did you forget to put it in there, too?

Surgeon: Yes. When I forget it once, I will forget it forever until that – for some reason or not something will shake my head and then I will recall.

Attorney: Fair enough. And nothing about Mr. Vaughan's course up to this point made you remember any of that?

Surgeon: No.

Attorney: Now, you have – it is your opinion that during this hospitalization from September 8th to September 27th that Mr. Vaughan was Dr. P***'s patient, he was the captain of the ship and you were just consulting?

Surgeon: It is not just my opinion. That is the fact.

Attorney: And even if Mr. Vaughan is in there because of surgical complications from a surgery you performed, he is the other guy's patient, not yours?

Surgeon: That is wrong. That is not true. I saw Mr. Vaughan practically every day even though he was under the surgery of Dr. P***.

Attorney: You saw him practically every day?

Surgeon: Yes, sir.

Attorney: You and other doctors were caring for Mr. Vaughan during that time?

Surgeon: The gastroenterologist. But his main doctor was Dr. P*** at that time.

Attorney: Doctor, isn't it true that you never told the gastroenterologist that Mr. Vaughan had necrotizing pancreatitis until September 27, 2004, the day he was transferred to Norfolk?

Surgeon: I did not tell the gastroenterologist even on that day he was on the floor after I dictated the summary and he asked me why and I told him then why I think he should be going.

Attorney: The doctors who were treating Mr. Vaughan for those three weeks while he had steadily gotten worse didn't need to know that he had necrotizing pancreatitis? … Doctor, let me show you another document and ask you if that is your transfer note.

Surgeon: Yes.

Attorney: And that was written in connection with the transfer of Mr. Vaughan from Southampton Memorial Hospital to Norfolk General Hospital?

Surgeon: Yes, sir.

Attorney: And that is a note that you write to sort of give the history and the reason why he is being transferred to another care facility?

Surgeon: That note is dictated so that when he gets to see Dr. Perry he knew what happened. This is the third hospital admission of Mr. Vaughan so I think it is just proper just to give him a good discharge summary or transfer summary that he can read when he gets there.

Attorney: So it is at this time that it is first written down by you that Mr. Vaughan had a dry, black, almost charcoal paper pancreas; right?

Surgeon: When I dictate a transfer summary, I always review the chart, see what happened in the past, look at the operative note, look at the operation, look at the — all what happened in the past. And that is when I noted – I forgot to mention that the rest of the pancreas is dry, black, charcoal paper. And that is when I dictated it.

Attorney: Okay. So you –

Surgeon: that is the first time I realized I was – I didn't even – it wasn't written in there.

Attorney: You forgot to put it in your op note, you forgot to put it in the discharge note, you forgot to put it in an admit consult; and, yet, you look back at this chart, you forgot every time and you look back at this chart that didn't have any mention of it in there and that chart reminded you that it should have been in there, is that what you are telling this jury?

Surgeon: Yes, sir. Yes, sir. I just forgot it.

Attorney: You want this jury to believe that, Doctor?

Surgeon's Attorney: Objection, Your Honor.

Court: Sustained.

Attorney: I am sorry. Withdraw that. Doctor, isn't it true that you were consulted on the 27th, you pulled out the mushroom catheter and a large amount of pus came out?

Surgeon: I am looking at the exact date when I pulled out that catheter. I was consulted on the 9th. Okay. On the 27th, I had pulled out the mushroom catheter, the tube. That is because it hasn't been draining any fluid for the past two or three days.

Attorney: What happened when you pulled it out?

Surgeon: Large amount of pus came out.

Attorney: And that – and that is the day you decided that he should go to Norfolk?

Surgeon: No. Three or four days before that is when I want him transferred.

Attorney: Where does it say in your notes that you wanted him transferred three or four days before?

Surgeon: No. No. It is not in the note. I told you, it is not my style to write something in there that doesn't – that the attending physician don't agree.

Attorney: So three or four days before, the attending physician and you agreed that he should be transferred?

Surgeon: No. No. I have told Dr. P*** three to four days before transfer that I think Mr. Vaughan should go to Norfolk General for a pancreatic debridement.

Attorney: But Dr. P*** didn't send him?

Surgeon: He didn't say anything.

Attorney: So you and he disagreed on that?

Surgeon: I don't know whether he disagreed or what. He just didn't say anything.

Attorney: But that didn't go into your notes?

Surgeon: I don't think I should write —- I don't want to write that. I didn't want to write that.

Attorney: So a few moments ago you told us that you don't put things in your notes that the doctors agree to; it is, you put in what the doctors disagree on?

Surgeon: I didn't say that. I don't put notes that we disagree. I put notes that we agree.

Attorney: Okay. So you disagreed – you and Dr. P*** disagreed that Mr. Vaughan should go to Norfolk three or four days before he went there, correct? You wanted him to go and Dr. P*** didn't or didn't say anything?

Surgeon: Incorrect. That is right. He didn't say anything.

Attorney: He didn't say anything?

Surgeon: That is right.

Attorney: And at this time, Doctor, weren't you concerned with Mr. Vaughan's wellbeing?

Surgeon: I was concerned three or four days before. That is why I told him I think we should get him transferred to Norfolk General.

Attorney: And you didn't do anything else except tell that to Dr. P***?

Surgeon: I don't know what else I can do.

Attorney: And, of course, your chart is silent on it, it doesn't say one way or the other. Doctor, isn't it true that you wrote on the transfer summary dated 9/27 that Mr. Vaughan's pancreas is dry, black almost charcoal paper?

Surgeon: I wrote that.

Attorney: Let me finish my question, sir.

Surgeon: Okay.

Attorney: Isn't it true that you wrote that on September 27th?

Surgeon: Yes, sir. That is true.

Attorney: Because you knew at the time that Mr. Vaughan was going to lose his pancreas?

Surgeon: No. No. No. That is not the reason. No. Let me finish.

Attorney: No, sir. You answer my question.

Surgeon: Let me finish.

Court: Stop. Let him ask the question. Allow him to answer the question without interruption.

Attorney: Yes, sir.

Court: You don't interrupt him and he won't interrupt you.

Surgeon: I hope so.

Court: Rephrase your question.

Attorney: You wrote for the first time on September 27th, that Mr. Vaughan's pancreas, back when you operated on him in August, was dry, black and charcoal paper because it was apparent to you on the 27th that Mr. Vaughan was going to lose his pancreas?

Surgeon: No.

Attorney: Okay. You have answered that question. And you wanted to make it look like that Mr. Vaughan was going to lose his pancreas all along?

Surgeon: No.

Attorney: That is not true?

Surgeon: No.

Attorney: Okay. Doctor, isn't it true that when you first had Mr. Vaughan as a patient and you went in and did whatever you did to the head of his pancreas in August that his pancreas was not infected?

Surgeon: Correct.

Attorney: And we can agree that by the time you were done with your care and treatment of Mr. Vaughan that his pancreas was very infected?

Surgeon: No. I don 't agree with that.

Attorney: You don't agree with that?

Surgeon: (Witness shaking head.)

Attorney: It was not infected on the 27th?

Surgeon: No. It was on the 27th. But that is at the time of –

Attorney: I am sorry.

Surgeon: It was on the 27th. So my – my notes around 23, around September 23, 24, I thought that is when I first state it is getting infected.

Attorney: So we can agree, can't we, that when you – when he started with you, he wasn't infected; when he finished with you, he was?

Surgeon: No. No. When he was infected on the 24th. Yes. Remember, I finished the operation way before that.

Attorney: Okay. So you don't consider yourself as being involved after that point?

Surgeon: No. What I am saying, there is no sign of active infection on the September 24, 23. Also I had mentioned before, he was getting better when he came in on the 17th – on the 9th and Dr. P*** agreed that he is getting better. He even signed off on the chart that he is not going to follow the patient anymore. And Dr. P*** dictated a discharge summary on the 10th. So after that point, he was getting better.

Attorney: And your discharge summary just happened to remember about that old, dead pancreas?

Surgeon: When I write a transfer summary, I want to give the receiving surgeon as much information as I can gather. And that is when I always review my operative note. And that is what I found out. I said, Lord, I didn't mention that the pancreas was dry, black, paper charcoal. And that is why I put that on the transfer note.

Attorney: Well, your attorney, in his opening remarks to the jury, said that you didn't put it in there initially because you weren't dealing with the pancreas. It is almost as if it wasn't really important. But is it important now on the transfer?

Surgeon: I didn't say it wasn't important. I said I forgot it.

He forgot. He forgot to tell his patient and his patient's doctors that he had just lost a major organ. His pancreas. An organ, that according to current medical literature, a body can't live without and medical science has no plan for someone to live without. The loss of this organ is so rare, if someone does lose it electively or not, the Centers for Disease Control and the National Center for Health Statistics don't even have statistics to show it.

No, we did not win the case. We did not receive any compensation for the organ the hospital contagion ate up after a surgical procedure that should never have happened in the first place. Virginia caps medical malpractice lawsuits, so we never did mention a figure to the jury and never could set a cost for our loss. But Shirley and I know the cost: it was our dream of a peaceful ending to our lives together. It was retirement savings flushed into an endless cycle of expenses to keep me alive that no one could have foreseen, like relocating to a cramped apartment and out of our beloved home and neighborhood that had become toxic to my body while we investigated the source – our neighbor's household trash burning incinerator.

Why did we lose the lawsuit? Who knows? Maybe that few times removed batch of small town jurors? I watched the judge as the clerk handed him the jury's decision to read. His eyes widened and he flippantly tossed the verdict to the clerk of court who caught it on the fly before it hit the floor.

A few days later, a nice young man who served as an alternate juror came to our home and told us he was sorry for the way the case had gone. He said he would have made sure things had turned out differently had they counted his vote. He was so sorry, he felt compelled to travel to our attorney's office and tell him this as well. We helped him relieve his conscience the best we could, but even he could not understand what had happened.

If you have never filed a medical malpractice lawsuit before, think twice and then again before you do. You are going to get the beating of your life on the stand, and so will the people you love. If you are not heirs to a fortune, you will need to work on a contingency with an attorney who has reviewed the case and is betting you will win before taking it. Your high stakes poker playing, hired gun will be facing a show down with well-groomed, well-paid card sharks on the pay role of insurance companies whose purpose in life is to make sure they don't pay no matter what. To keep going with this analogy, the deck will be stacked against you from the outset. Shirley and I were accused of all kinds of hooey, directly and indirectly. Implied allegations are lawyers' fortes and get jurors distracted into details that detract from the obvious, like a surgeon didn't remember to mention to anyone that a man's body he opened up supposedly had a dead organ in it.

Shirley and I were chastised like children on the court witness stand by the surgeon's attorneys that we should have known there were risks to surgery. Didn't I know that? Looking back, I freely admit this: I did not know that I needed to research the variety of risks and adverse outcomes of a common gallbladder surgery or what the medical community refers to as the "standard of care". Yes, I was suffering debilitating pain and ordered to have surgery for gallbladder removal, but really, in the meantime, according to the finger-wagging card sharks, I should have dismissed my surgeon's diagnosis, appointed myself and Shirley as my own researchers and doctors, second-guessed his recommendations, and taken a crash course in endocrinology.

And here it is in plain language. Here is the quandary of modern medicine: it does some pretty nifty things when you need it, but if you are really sick and not able to become your own science researcher and patient advocate, you might later be blamed for trusting the doctor, hospital and medical system and for not finding out the truth of your condition for yourself, including possible complications, side effects and life-altering scenarios. You might be blamed, as I was blamed by the surgeon's defense attorney while sitting in a witness stand four years after I "lost" my pancreas, for not doing your homework while simultaneously being debilitated by sickness. We hope the resource section in the back of this book will help you become a savvier consumer of medical services than we were in 2004. Now we know.

Why did we lose a lawsuit when the doctor's only defense was that he "forgot"? My money is on the last century beef with the family cow.

CHAPTER FIVE:

A Canary In A Coalmine

"There's so much pollution in the air now that if it weren't
for our lungs there'd be no place to put it all."

—Robert Orben

Of the many roles Shirley assumed in 2004, one of the most
important has been the Chronicler of our Daily Lives. Had it
not been for the detailed logs of my blood glucose levels and our
daily activities, we may not have ever solved the mystery of my on
and off again "flu" that would last for a few days and then disap-
pear like the morning mist — which, did in fact, have something
to do with the mystery illnesses.

If the University of Verona, Italy, study of May 2010 is any
indication of medical trends, there may be more people learning
to live without a pancreas in the future, and of those people, many
of them may not know how daily life will affect them until they
are worn down from it and wondering, what happened? Here is
something that may happen: you may find yourself sensitive to
environmental toxins that are so prevalent in modern life that you
won't be able to see the forest for the trees when you find yourself
asking, "Why can't I get my blood glucose levels down? What's
wrong with me?"

It took a while, almost a year, before we figured out the cause of my recurring mystery illness. Our very first outing after the surgery and long winter was to our daughter's home in the spring. This first trip began with an inventory and packing of everything that was going to be needed to travel the short distance, but may as well have been a trip to Mars. The creation of the life-saving, day-tripping briefcase began with everything from lists of medications, lists of doctors, logs of insulin and blood sugar readings, two glucometers, extra lancets and strips, an extra insulin pump and its ice pick attachments, needles, insulin bottles, enzymes, emergency contact lists, and combination locks on the case to make sure we would not be ticketed for transporting drug paraphernalia if a police officer pulled us over. The emptied out, half gallon, plastic white vinegar jug did not fit in the case. It was used to collect any "bio-hazard" materials, like needles, that would then be dropped off at the local clinic. The clinic instructed us to make sure there were no shreds of paper with our names and address on them accidentally disposed of into the jug, as they believed and told us, "drug addicts in the clinic's lobby might find out where you live and break into your house for the needles." Not really sure why they believed this, since anyone can buy needles without a prescription, but we complied with their instructions anyway.

The three day trip to Shirley's daughter's home in North Carolina revealed what we had suspected: something in our home or around our home was making it difficult and sometimes impossible to keep my blood glucose levels below 200, and sometimes even 300. The three days in North Carolina were "easy" compared to our usual frantic battles to monitor and adjust, monitor and adjust. My blood glucose stayed down and the haze around my own mind and flu-like symptoms left.

We returned home more determined than ever to repeat the optimum blood glucose levels. Our logs were invaluable. Eventually a pattern and relationship emerged of waking up with our neighborhood enveloped in a heavy smoke that hung low to the ground and my elevated blood glucose followed by predictable days of flu-like illness. We only had to look across the connecting backyards of our neighborhood to spy the source of the smoke. The culprit was a neighbor who had recently installed an outdoor wood-burning stove, but instead of burning approved wood or wood chips, the cheapskate would try to save himself a trip to the dump by burning his household trash in the burner – plastics and all.

Not ready to go back to the nights of little sleep now that we knew the source of the problem, Shirley decided to make a logical and friendly appeal to the neighbor. She set out across the yard to knock on his front door on a morning when the evidence could accompany her – the low-lying cloud of toxic smoke poured from the blazing outdoor wood stove's exhaust pipe. She politely shared with him our problems with the smoke, that I was doing my best to live without a pancreas, and that the smoke was making my blood glucose levels uncontrollable. In a Christian way, she asked the neighbor to please stop burning the household trash at least, if not all burning, if he could manage it. In a not-so-Christian way, she was told to buzz off, except not that four letter word. To her credit, Shirley knew a foot stomping dance would be wasted on this person's front door steps, so she just turned and walked the 160 feet back home.

The burning days and smoky mornings almost seemed to intensify after that, so much so, Shirley could not keep my blood glucose levels down and I couldn't take the flu-like symptoms anymore. Then summer really hit and the Virginia heat and humidity prevented most people from spending too much time outside for any activity, and certainly not burning trash. The fall saw a few smoky mornings, but then, for whatever reason, maybe it was the economy driving the guy to pinch pennies on curb pick-up for the trash or a dump run, but the smoke-filled neighborhood became unbearable and we knew we could not stay. In the winters of 2007, 2008 and 2009, we left our home, with the boxwood maze the grandchildren loved, and our memories from our lifetime together, and moved into a cramped apartment in the neighboring city of Franklin.

By this time, we had added a new member to our family. In 2006, after two years of successfully solving the case of the missing pancreas — well, successful because I was alive — we decided to celebrate and bring a sweet, little eight-week old puppy into our family. Maybe for most people our age a puppy isn't such a good idea, but we were already up all night, so training and caring for a puppy, whose body clock was as full on as our glucose testing clock, was no problem. Sir Bentley, a registered standard Chihuahua we almost named Diamond Jack after the two prominent white diamonds on his neck, turned out to be a needed, bright spot in our lives and valuable member of our diabetes management team.

As Sir Bentley grew up, a sixth doggy sense seemed to turn on for him as if he knew something wasn't quite right with me. He preferred to sleep in my bed, and Shirley and I noticed, as we had trained ourselves to notice everything coming and going, that he seemed to know when I was in danger of an insulin reaction, a severe, life-threatening drop in my blood glucose level. Sir Bentley would lick me during the beginning of these drops, and then push me with his head until I woke up. If all else failed, his attempts to rouse me would escalate into barking. Shirley speculates that he smells something different that doesn't set right with him, perhaps coming through my skin as my blood glucose tanks. We don't know, but our steadfast little guy's ability to serve as backup for Shirley and I brought us a little more peace of mind, especially during the night.

Lest you think we were overly anxious about this outdoor wood burning stove issue, you should know that the smoke from the stove was so thick on occasions, that the health care center about three blocks from us called the fire department to investigate the source of the smoke and relocated their patients temporarily. There was enough anger about the smoke from enough neighbors that we decided to post some flyers and circulate a petition to demand the town council ban the outdoor wood-burning stoves – all TWO of them, as we found out. And here is where the small town fun began.

The other OWB stove, as a town council member informed us when we and the petitioner friends gathered to face our town council members, belonged to the mayor's son. In a show of political solidarity, our town council members could not see their way to banning the OWBS when one of two of the town stoves belonged to our revered mayor's son.

Perhaps logic, science and a reference to the town's written history wasn't the tack to take with this crew. At the meeting in August 2007, we petitioners pointed out that the town had experienced a similar issue in 1950, when the town adopted an ordinance to eliminate the menacing smoke cloud hanging over our streets and homes by shutting down all of the smokehouses within the town's limits. We pointed out that these old-fashioned smoke houses contained far fewer pollutants and citizens were limited in exposure to about 200 smoke hours per year.

Shirley and I presented our mounting expenses for having to take a temporary residence in the neighboring city during the heavy burning months of fall and winter. I tried to appeal to my town council members by reminding them of what they already knew about me, that I was a sharecropper's son who had grown up in substandard housing, if you could call it that. Didn't I deserve to be able to live in the home I built for my family in 1964? Didn't I deserve to be able to open the windows of my house and not get sick from toxic smoke filling my home? We tried to read their faces to see if there was a sense of sympathy and doing the right thing growing, but it was futile. The unspoken political bond to protect the offspring of their fearless leader, the town mayor, appeared to be overriding common sense.

And then one free-thinker broke from the pack and offered this earth-shattering insight, "Mr. Vaughan, if we ban outdoor wood-burning stoves, we will have to ban all the town barbeques and grills as well! They make smoke, too!"

"Yes," I confirmed. "Grills do smoke, but OWBS are outlawed in many other states and counties for their known ill health effects, especially when household trash is burned in them. When they are used, they must be 500 feet and downwind from any other human. This one is 160 feet from my back door." And this is where we probably lost them – when we introduced the science.

Having worked as a lab analyst at a chemical company for 40 years, I knew a little something about the serious health effects of plastics broken down by heat and dispersed through the air and into the unprotected tissues of your nasal passages and lungs. I also knew the constantly running ventilation and exhaust system in the chemical company where I worked were there for a reason. I shared with the bleary-eyed council members the simple fact: open burning creates dioxin – one of humankind's most toxic chemicals – the same harmful chemical contained in Agent Orange – you know, Vietnam? No bells.

I continued. Dioxin contamination lasts for years in our environment. It accumulates in our fat cells where it can build up to toxic levels. As I scanned the hefty row of council members that last fact struck home with me and I considered I'd hit on a reason for the lack of intelligent response to our petition. But I pressed on with our citizens' duty.

I read off a quote that seemed to sum up the threat of OWBS trash burning, "A recent study found that residential trash burning from a single home could release more dioxin into the air than an industrial incinerator with thousands of customers." [1] I paused for effect. Nothing. So I continued.

Many states have outlawed outdoor burning of trash for a reason. Trash today is not the same as it was years ago. Today's trash contains plastics, metals and other synthetic materials. When burned in a burn barrel, woodstove, fireplace, or open fire these items emit toxic fumes and harmful quantities of dioxins, a group of highly toxic chemicals known to cause cancer, asthma and other illnesses. Typically, dioxins do not exist in materials before they are incinerated, but are produced when waste is burned. Significantly higher levels of dioxins are created by burning trash in rural settings than in municipal incinerators. Household burning receives limited oxygen, and thus burn at fairly low temperatures, producing not only dioxins, but a great deal of smoke and other pollutants. Unlike the stoves and barrels used in backyard burning, large incinerators are required by EPA regulations to have stringent pollution control systems that reduce dioxin emissions primarily by preventing their formation. Backyard burning is also particularly dangerous because it releases pollutants at ground level where they are more readily inhaled or incorporated into the food chain. [2]

HERE ARE THE KNOWN FACTS ABOUT OUTDOOR TRASH BURNING:

- Emissions from backyard burning of household trash can increase the risk of heart disease; aggravate respiratory ailments such as asthma; cause rashes, nausea, or headaches, and developmental or reproductive disorders. Over time, exposure to these toxic chemicals can lead to chronic diseases such as emphysema and cancer

- Toxins and other pollutants from trash burning affect everyone's health and property. The toxins released into the air can enter your body through your eyes, protective mucous in your nose, or through blood vessels in your lungs.

- Trash burning occurs at low temperatures in burn barrels, homemade burn boxes, wood stoves, outdoor boilers, or open pits and lacks pollution controls. Large modern incinerators burn at over 1800 degrees and add enough oxygen for complete combustion. These very hot fires destroy some of the dangerous chemicals otherwise produced by backyard burning. Sophisticated pollution control devices capture other toxins or pollutants.

- One half of the health risks associated with trash burning are a direct result of smoke inhalation. The other half occur when toxic particles are deposited in water, soils, crops and gardens and then ingested.

- Children are especially at risk because their immune systems are not fully developed. A child breathing the same polluted air as an adult will absorb up to six times more of the combustion products per body weight. [3]

The amount of information online to help us get our point across about the seriousness of backyard trash burning was substantial and easily available to anyone who cared to look. There were even great graphs, like the one above, that our tax dollars had paid for us to use. This graph is interesting because it shows that while municipal waste and hazardous waste incineration decreased from 1987 to 2000, backyard garbage burning barely declined. The statistic made me wonder if all local ordinance regulators were as unmovable as the line-up I faced.

The EPA's educational tools encouraged citizens to "Check to see what type of burning laws your local area has and who enforces these laws" and then to "Work with your local government to pass either burn ban laws or a burn ban resolution." [5] I would like to have the guy who wrote that recommendation come to my town anytime he likes, I thought.

The EPA online "community education toolkit" didn't leave me high and dry. Its final recommendation was: if you educate the children of the community through the school system on the dangers of backyard burning you can then expect, "Decreased burning due to children influencing parental decisions." I tried to imagine the kid next door with the smoke pouring through his window in the middle of the night from his own homegrown burning experiment asking his parents to cool it with their Agent Orange release program. Right.

While we regaled the town council with science, I really wished I could find materials from the EPA's website that may have been more suitable to the audience at the petitioners' meeting. The EPA's website offered childlike programs featuring Bernie the Burn Barrel, a "reformed burner", but no Woody the Wood Stove. I was out of luck.

The council dismissed the petition, and with it common sense, a mountain of science and any hope of a peaceful winter in our home for Shirley and I.

A few days after the petition and our citizens' complaints were dismissed, a sympathetic town councilman stopped by my home and confessed to me in our front yard that he would like to shut down the stove. "But it's not the stove that's the problem, you know," he leaned into make his point. "It's the owner that's the problem."

I didn't know what he meant by this revelation, but I did appreciate his willingness to share his sympathy and insights. I shared his secret with Shirley and between the two of us - who were staring at another winter in a spider-infested city apartment - we decided to make appearances at the town council meetings every time they opened the door.

After a while, they saw us coming and got out their alarm clocks – which they used to restrict our presentation to a five-minute time limit. Fine, I thought. I won't bother to regale them with tax-payer sponsored science reports any idiot can find right on the internet. I covered the basics of our complaint, for the record and with the clock ticking, and worked my way up to my new information.

"I think we've covered the science supporting our complaint many times by now. And I know you know this is solid and we are in our right to ask for you to use your authority to protect us in our own home. In fact, I would like to repeat the conversation I had with one of you on my front lawn…"

"Your time is UP, MR. VAUGHAN!" shouted the council chairwoman.

You would have thought we were on the verge of betraying state secrets or launching a real grenade instead of an inquiry that would just serve to fracture their appearance of solidarity on the issue. The councilwoman not only yelled that our time was up, but motioned for the sergeant-at-arms to escort us from the room. As we were hustled toward the door, I took one look at the man's face in uniform and flashed on a late night memory of his patrol car pulling slowly down our lane toward the woman's home at the end of the street who seemed to be awfully popular. Why watch reality shows for entertainment when you can live in a small town? I thought, the unasked question for the town councilman still stuck in my throat behind my gaping mouth.

The escalation after this town meeting was ugly. The burning intensified and we began looking for a less buggy apartment to move to for the winter months. I know, I probably shouldn't have snapped, but early on a Sunday morning thick with smoke outside our windows, I watched Shirley sitting on the sofa rocking in pain from a migraine and thought of the hell of the coming days of my flu-like symptoms and the effect it would have on my blood glucose and, well, I picked up the phone and called the mayor at home.

I don't mind admitting it; I had cracked up by this time and would like to blame it on the toxins and the strain. But it was really that I had come to the end of my rope. I told the town mayor I didn't care if his son owned one of those blame stoves, the one behind my home was making my wife and I sick and it had to go. I may have even said something like, "if this doesn't get resolved and fast, there's going to be bloodshed!"

The prompt letter addressed to my home from the town attorney came to the point: "…in my opinion, the Town is not in position to take any action with respect to your neighbor's wood-burning furnace. It does not amount to a public nuisance. Although you have been advised of the Town's position, you insist on pressing the issue. This past Sunday morning, you called the Mayor at his home very early about this matter. In the course of that conversation, you made remarks that were threatening in nature. Such action will not be tolerated by the Mayor or the Town Council. Cease and desist from any such statements or actions in the future."

In 2008, out of shear desperation and in genuine despair, we decided to put our beloved family home up for sale. When the realtor dropped by one morning to hammer the sign in the ground, the burning was full on and our neighborhood looked like the mystical isle of Brigadoon could be hiding just beyond the next misty, tree-lined lane.

"Is it like this all the time?" the new realtor asked, looking around and pointing out the fog, like we'd never seen this phenomenon. So we shrugged and tried to look innocent. "You're not going to be able to sell this place if it is."

He was right. Between the stock market bottoming out in 2008 and the menace of the morning mist, our home sat flat for a year.

After a year of rolling past the tall pines and for sale sign in the front yard, going back and forth between another buggy, city apartment and the comfortable home we wished we could live in,

The summer we were finishing up this book, CNN aired its *Toxic America* series with Dr. Sanjay Gupta and its tagline, "Toxic America: It could be your town. It could be your childhood." [9] We felt a little gleeful with the mountain of validation the splashy and lengthy, investigative series gave our little, small town crusade. Just as we found there are a lot of people working together to help patients become aware and empowered to avoid becoming a hospital safety statistic, there were also many people, millions, who were finding out how modern chemicals were affecting our country's health and were willing to risk social or political ridicule to do something about it.

We didn't feel gleeful at all about the President's Council report that also came out in the summer of 2010 stating some 41 percent of Americans will be diagnosed with cancer at some point in their lives. The President's Cancer Panel released a landmark 200-page report in the beginning of May of 2010 calling on Americans to "rethink the way we confront cancer, including much more rigorous regulation of chemicals."

We went from feeling gleeful and vindicated to a little sheepish with the way the issue of modern chemicals and health picked up steam that summer. We heard the television news announce the new bill in Congress called the Safer Chemicals Act of 2010, an ambitious bill aimed at revamping the 34-year-old Toxic Substances Control Act of 1976.

"This is not the first time Congress has attempted to fix our nation's flawed system for regulating toxic chemicals, but it is the first time that both chemical industry lobbyists and public health advocates agree that we can't delay change any longer — the scientific evidence is too overwhelming; the public outcry too loud" (save our town council), says the Safer Chemicals, Healthier families coalition on their website. The coalition represents more than

11 million individuals and includes parents, health professionals, advocates for people with learning and developmental disabilities, reproductive health advocates, environmentalists and businesses from across the nation. [10] That's right, businesses. That safer chemicals are good business should be common sense, so don't let anyone tell you it's one or the other. It can be both.

Why would chemical contaminants have such an effect on my blood glucose levels? What did the pancreas do that allowed me to live with so many invisible toxins before I lost it? I wish I knew. I hope someone is studying this, but as there are so few people being tracked who are living without a pancreas, I don't know if we will ever find out. What I do know is Sir Bentley and Shirley and I have had more restful nights and healthier days since we cleaned up our home and neighborhood. (And better church services.)

BASIC INGREDIENTS FOR NON-TOXIC CLEANER RECIPES

Five basic ingredients serve as the building blocks for many safe home cleaning needs:

1. *Baking Soda-* Cleans and deodorizes. Softens water to increase sudsing and cleaning power of soap. Good scouring powder.

2. *Borax -* Cleans and deodorizes. Excellent disinfectant. Softens water. Available in laundry section of grocery store.

3. *Soap-* Biodegrades safely and completely and is non-toxic. Available in grocery stores and health food stores. Sold as liquid, flakes, powder or in bars. Bars can be grated to dissolve more easily in hot water. Insist on soap without synthetic scents, colors or other additives.

4. *Washing Soda*- Cuts grease and removes stains. Disinfects. Softens water. Available in laundry section of grocery store or in pure form from chemical supply houses as "sodium carbonate."

5. *White Vinegar or Lemon Juice* - Cuts grease and freshens.

HOUSEHOLD CLEANER

Mix together:

    1 tsp. liquid soap (castile, peppermint)
    1 tsp. borax
    Squeeze of lemon
    1 quart warm water

    OR

    ¼ cup baking soda
    ½ cup borax
    ½ cup vinegar
    1 gallon water

CHAPTER SIX:

What Happened to Food?

"As a culture we seem to have arrived at a place where whatever native wisdom we may once have possessed about eating has been replaced by confusion and anxiety... How did we ever get to a point where we need investigative journalists to tell us where our food comes from and nutritionists to determine the dinner menu?"

—- Michael Pollan,
The Omnivore's Dilemma:
The Natural History of Four Meals

I thought I knew what food was. Where it came from, how it got here, and what it looked like on a plate. So it shouldn't have been so surprising, upon reflection, that learning to eat without my pancreas would be a journey that would lead me back to knowledge I gleaned in childhood: Good food comes from good soil and the quicker you eat it after it is taken from the soil, the better it is for you.

By the time I was six years-old, my father put a hoe in my hand and the hand of my twin brother, Carl, and took us out to the fields to grow one of the many abundant crops that sprang from the fertile soils of Southeastern Virginia. As a sharecropper's son, we rotated through different fields, crops and farms depending upon the season and the work availability. I also rotated through different high schools, as was normal for farming families back then, but I did manage to graduate in 1950.

Of the fields, farms and crops that I tended with my family during my childhood and adolescence, the one crop we knew the most intimately was peanuts. People looking for peanuts in specialty and gourmet shops know Virginia peanuts are the highest quality on the market. The sandy soil in Southeastern Virginia is perfect for the crop, which has been grown here since 1840s and was brought to this region from Africa by enslaved Africans, although it is a native of South America. Spanish conquistadores exploring the New World found South American Indians eating what many called cacohuate, or "earth cocoa" and then gradually exported and transplanted the plant to West Africa.[1]

The versatile, tasty morsel we call the peanut is the pod or legume of the arachis hypogea plant, a member of the same botanical family as the ordinary green pea. But the peanut is an unusual member of the pea family, since its pods have the peculiar habit of ripening underground. [2]

My memories of standing in acres of sandy fields surrounded by woods displaying fall's colorful glory and harvesting peanuts is so engrained in my mind, I commissioned a Virginian artist to paint a portrait of this vision of my family in our natural habitat. The painting hangs on the wall in the den of our home now. In the painting, my twin brother, Carl, and I are moving peanut plants that have been taken down from the "shocks," long stakes where they are piled in the field after they are uprooted, until we bring the red peanut picker to them for sorting into burlap bags.

In the painting, I am in the background, and the fact that I am holding my pitch fork with my right hand is a clue that this figure is me. Carl is behind the running peanut picker, and the fact that he is left-handed is also a dead giveaway that the figure is him pitching a forkful into the picker. That's not a smear in the middle of the painting, it is smoke and dust blowing from the peanut picker – an amazing piece of equipment invented by Benjamin F. Hicks, an African-American/Native American who received a patent for the machine in 1901 and lived in my county. Hicks' invention of the peanut picker is said to have revolution-ized farming in the area. A marker honoring his contribution to agriculture was erected near his farm by the Southampton Historical Society in 1988.[3]

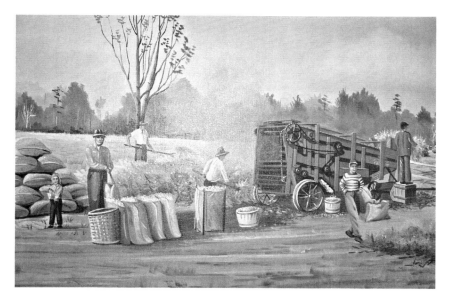

Detail of the painting of Clyde Vaughan's family.

My father stands where I still remember him, at the back of the picker using the ten inch long peanut needle to sew up the burlap bags with "ears" left on the corners so they could be picked up, stacked and transported to wherever they were headed, as all of the peanuts went out in time for Christmas. The artist painted my little brother, Richard, as walking away with his hands in his pockets. We teased him later and said the artist must have known him personally to capture his personality because he was always trying to get out of working. This wasn't really true, as he was usually caught up helping my mother with the younger children. My little sister took one look at the painting and was mortified that anyone would depict her with a *doll* in her arms. She's right, she didn't play with them. In fact, what you see in this painting is a picture of our family working *and* playing together. This is what we did to survive and how well we worked together was our relief from working so hard.

In most school classrooms, as soon as you mention peanuts the story of George Washington Carver and his many peanut inventions surface. As the National Peanut Board says of Carver, "It's not overstating matters to say that Dr. Carver and the peanut helped save the economy of the South." However, peanut butter is one peanut derivative we can't thank George Washington Carver for. That great favorite of the schoolboy was introduced by a St. Louis doctor in 1890 for patients who needed an easily digestible form of protein. As a food, peanuts are one of the most concentrated sources of nourishment known to man. Pound for pound, the peanut provides more protein, minerals, and vitamins than beef liver, more fat than heavy cream, and, dieters beware, more calories than sugar. [4]

And sometimes that protein isn't all peanut! The US Food and Drug Administration's guidelines for acceptable levels of insect parts in common foods allow for a regular size jar of peanut butter to legally contain up to 210 insect fragments before it's officially declared unsanitary! Mark my words, school kids will and probably do know that and will still eat and love peanut butter.

As a sharecropper's son, I am not one of those people who will ever regale you with stories of "the good old days." Life was hard when I was growing up, even harsh. The availability of food, especially, is fascinating to me. I look around at people literally "running" through drive-thru windows and Wal-Marts now and think, very few people know how hard life used to be for most families living right here in our county.

When I graduated from high school, I had spent so much of my youth expending the few calories I ate on hard physical labor I weighed only 102 pounds. Over the next few years of my life, as I took a job at the local chemical company as a lab analyst, I was able to afford to buy more food for myself, and not expend those calories so quickly. In those first few years after high school, I finally got the calories I needed to finish growing and shot up from a lanky 5' 2" to my full height and weight now, at 5' 10" and 168 pounds - eight inches in a handful of years. Shirley and I are both proud of the fact that we can still fit into our wedding clothes, 40 years later.

What happened to food? It really isn't a mystery, and if you think it is, you need only spend an afternoon at the Southampton Heritage Village and Agriculture/Forestry Museum to solve the mystery.

The village and museum, two blocks from my home, is located on 10 acres of land and features small, original buildings moved from different parts of the county to a semi-circle around a grassy lawn. Among the small buildings is the original Wal-Mart: a country store with many of its original retail items, including five cent candy bars, medicines, and eerily enough, a children's coffin. Their brochure states the country store "had everything a farming family needed." When the county switched from horses to horse powered engines the country store became the gas station.

Other original buildings featured in the small village are a doctor/dentist office (because they were the same profession back then), a one room schoolhouse, a two-room country dwelling, chicken house, ice house, blacksmith shop, outhouse and a pig pen. The tavern where my great-great-great grandfather's niece became the last victim in the Southampton Insurrection now stands opposite the village in a field with a sign noting "The Rebecca Vaughan House".

Three warehouse-sized buildings across the gravel parking lot from the village surround a covered area with picnic tables, where volunteers will offer you a cold Coke and an hour long tour for only three dollars. The village and museum are open three days a week for four hours at a time. This is not a fancy, glass-cased and parquet floor museum, but the over 7,000 collected items from our county's rural history displayed proudly on donated or handmade tables, right where you can see and touch them, represent something priceless, something many people are beginning to wonder about and question as the economy tanks and we're all realizing something is going to need to change... Taken as a whole and as portal to the not so distant past, to the aware visitor, the museum presents the collective wisdom and truth of what a community who knows how to take care of itself, its soil, its animals, and each other, looks like. Or, looked like.

The museum tour starts at the beginning of agricultural history with the authentic tools Native American's used to harvest and prepare plants and animals from the local woods and fields. There are dozens of stone mortar and pestles and hundreds of different sizes and shapes of arrow heads. There are ancient wood-working and farming tools used by settlers, and as you proceed down an aisle with walls lined with sharp implements and tables littered with hand carved equipment whose uses you can only guess (the volunteer will tell you, of course) what you will notice is the increased mechanization and complexity of the tools developed for growing food as times changed. The wooden plows, originally compact and sturdy digging sticks, become larger and more cumbersome with added leather harnessing to attach to animals and metal points to cut through the soil. In the most advanced plows, a harrow is added to turn the soil, not just dig a row to plant seeds; but as fast as you are taking in and deciphering the uses of these daily farming tools, POW! You turn a corner and spot your first John Deere tractor! The tractor. Reverent pause here. The collection of children's toy tractors in the museum alone – donated from a single patron's collection - is worth the price of admission.

The tractors get bigger as you go down another aisle and you wish you could sit on one, bounce up and down and make a motoring sound with pursed lips as, today, they are associated with toys and playing. There are so many varieties and styles of peanut pickers, you realize a lot of people had the same idea about the same time in making so many versions of the revolutionary machine. By the time you're getting tired, and might think it's time to go, you'd be wrong, because now you are going to learn about trucks and trains and the two warehouses full of gas powered vehicles leading us up to the middle of the last century. As you cross the lawn to the next warehouse, you will pass two Goliath sized millstones – that sit silent until the mules are brought in used to grind corn for meal on the museum's Heritage Day Festivals in September.

About the time you feel worn out, you'll remember the display you saw earlier, in the first warehouse, of the social meeting area for rural families in the early 1900s, a recreated back porch, and you'd be thinking about the necessity of having one of those to sit on at the end of a day of hooking up animals to plows, or riding a real John Deere, or loading a truck full of peanuts to ship to a market further up North in time for Christmas. The recreated farm house kitchen would also be a necessity for sitting with your family at the end of the day and thanking the Lord for the good food you are now going to share.

The mystery of what happened to food will be solved by the time you leave the museum, if you don't forget that you are not visiting a quantum physics lab. What happened during your wandering and wondering through the time portal aisles? Did the times change or did time itself change? Did the days get shorter in the last one hundred years? Or did the machines that we use to live get faster and faster and faster? And, because the museum isn't about the faceless industry of modern agri-business that continues to replace family farms in America, you didn't even get to see the combine they import from China these days to do all the work in the fields!

Like everyone else who grew up during the industrial agri-business' takeover of food production in the twentieth century, I appreciated, probably more than some, the ability to leave behind me and all human beings the back-breaking, never-ending work of growing food. But something happened between the first time a farmer happily jumped on his first John Deere to grow food in local fields that were cared for like children, for local families, and today, when food is imported from an average of 1500 miles before it reaches our overflowing store shelves. In fact, the average carrot travels 1,828 miles from the farm to the table where it is eaten, according to the Leopold Center for Sustainable Agriculture's July 2003 report. [5]

Here's where I could write a whole other book on corporate farming, government subsidies, and the pesticides and herbicides used to force plants into producing yields beyond any 20th century farmer's wildest dreams while stripping the soil and its dependent crops – our food - of most real nutrients. I could go on and on about how most of America's major crops, like corn, end up being converted into a high-fructose corn syrup food substance that is now being blamed for the epidemic of diabetes and obesity, and how fructose specifically acts like jet-fuel for pancreatic tumors, according to a University of California 2010 study.[6] But instead, I will defer to the dozens of books already written on this subject and just say this, what passes for food today, isn't allowed to pass through my body now that I am living without my pancreas.

Remember the research frenzy I went through to present our case against the backyard burning for our town council? Along the way, I discovered it wasn't just the cleaners I needed to watch out for if I was going to keep my insulin effective and my blood glucose under control. There were also concerns, as that same President's Cancer Panel in 2010 revealed, with food. All kinds in every modern processed and packaged can and box lining store shelves in every town and city across the country.

The President's Cancer Panel suggested to Americans, if they wanted to decrease their 41 percent chance of getting cancer, that they eat whole food, meaning food that was not coated with pesticides and herbicides and not run through a factory and put into a box. There was a name for this kind of food: organic. That name is so associated with hippies and people from California, I and a lot of people weren't happy about it. I think there's a different word, one that makes sense where I come from and that word is *traditional*.

Looking around at the museum, you don't see displayed tanks of pesticides and herbicides or a celebration involving mules and a grindstone to distribute processed corn syrup. Did all of this chemical warfare on food happened sometime after the museum's timeline ended and the last exhibit left off with the happy tractors and revolutionary peanut pickers? Taking in the white-washed, simple buildings that comprised the Heritage Village of the museum, another thought occurred to me. What if people used to be better at policing what when into their own food because they were a part of the process? A part of a community that knew each other and knew where their food came from?

In his investigation of the question, "What should we have for dinner?" Michael Pollan, an investigative journalist, wrote the book *The Omnivore's Dilemma: A Natural History of Four Meals* in 2006. In the *New York Times* bestseller, Pollan postulates that America "as a relatively new nation" and its hodge-podge of "immigrant populations" were unable to resist the takeover of family farms and proliferation of industrially processed food without "a single, strong, stable culinary tradition to guide us."

"The lack of a steadying culture of food leaves us especially vulnerable to the blandishments of the food scientist and the marketer... It is very much in the interest of the food industry to exacerbate our anxieties about what to eat, the better to then assuage them with new products," write Pollan in the introduction to The Omnivore's Dilemma. "Our bewilderment in the supermarket is no accident."

In the era represented by the museum, people definitely knew where their food originated, and probably that farmer's family line back to Moses. From the canning equipment on display in the museum, to cider presses and the ice house and smoke house in the village circle, it appeared that families took part in preserving their own food. I know this is true. Because growing up, my family did this as well.

Maybe by the time you leave the museum, you too will have the burning question in your mind of What Happened to Food? If you really want to know what happened after the days of local family farms in America - who is growing your food now, where is it being grown and how is it being grown - you can find out in the documentary *Food, Inc.* In the popular documentary (it was the number one selling DVD in 2010) filmmaker Robert Kenner "lifts the veil on our nation's food industry, exposing the highly mechanized underbelly that has been hidden from the American consumer with the consent of our government's regulatory agencies, USDA and FDA."[7]

Be prepared to lose your appetite as the documentary, and its website, answer: "Our nation's food supply is now controlled by a handful of corporations that often put profit ahead of consumer health, the livelihood of the American farmer, the safety of workers and our own environment. We have bigger-breasted chickens, the perfect pork chop, herbicide-resistant soybean seeds, even tomatoes that won't go bad, but we also have new strains of E. coli—the harmful bacteria that causes illness for an estimated 73,000 Americans annually. We are riddled with widespread obesity, particularly among children, and an epidemic level of diabetes among adults."

By the time you finish watching *Food, Inc*, you will probably want to visit the Southampton Village and Museum to see for yourself how food-growing was done before agri-business strategically killed American family farms and farming communities.

(I bet once the word gets out about the treasures they hold, the museum will need to increase its hours.)

Why is it important to know the answer to What Happened to Food? Because you will then understand why the Standard American Diet, S.A.D., is killing us. "It's no mistake that the acronym for the Standard American Diet is S.A.D. When America exports the dietary principles of S.A.D. to another country, a decline in the health of its people quickly follows. It also holds true for foreigners who immigrate here, as they quickly find out that their health declines and their weight increases when eating as the natives do. In all fairness, America should have signs at its entry borders that warn of the risks that go with adopting our S.A.D. lifestyle," says Dr. Jeffrey S. McCombs.[8]

In our ongoing experiments with foods my body would and would not accept, it was a no-brainer to think about food and what was going to work, not based on some philosophy, but on the hard data presented to us in our logs and records. My life depended upon us observing what foods improved my health and what foods did not. So how food was grown was a problem to be considered. But what about how it was packaged and canned?

When the FDA released its report cautioning consumers about the BPA lining cans and packages of even the healthiest foods, we weren't as stunned as the media wanted us to be.[9] In a 2010 independent study, aptly named *No Silver Lining*, another link, this time from packaging, to chronic disease and processed food was revealed.

"The FDA now says bisphenol A, BPA, the endocrine-disrupting, heart disease–causing ingredient in plastic food packaging and can linings, is not safe. Eating common canned foods is exposing consumers to levels of BPA equal to levels shown to cause health problems in laboratory animals," states the study that

am ostracized by my some of my neighbors and friends, and even members of my church, where I have attended for nearly half a century and since Richard Nixon was president. I am now a recognized and labeled rabble-rousing trouble-maker and given a social lashing via emails.

My own efforts to investigate and solve the mystery of my flu-like illness — that was relieved only by moving out of my mist-shrouded home into a newlywed apartment with giant spiders that didn't leave Shirley feeling quite like a newlywed — led me down a rabbit-hole called the internet and into a world of too-much-information. After applying my background as a senior lab analyst to sorting through endless research documents and reports, I concede the source of the on and off sickness lines up with our written records of blood glucose levels and burning days. But this information leads me to more and more levels of aware-ness that prompt us to look at our lives differently and in light of a the new context of modern life: chemicals aren't just belching out of my neighbor's outdoor wood burning stove, they are now in household products and the lining of food cans. In fact, to find food at all that is not coated in pesticides and herbicides is now a national pastime for a new species of health nuts who buy local, organic food and call themselves "locavores".

The level of awareness that I ascended to with the loss of my pancreas, and the life or death need to figure out how to live with-out it, provided me with the impetus for an education that I most likely would not have sought out otherwise. "A little learning is a dangerous thing," Thomas Jefferson said. Or a life-saving thing, I say.

While moving out of my home to avoid my neighbor's toxic ground cloud, I calculate that we are going to need to pay for my new existence for a long time and perhaps we should see an attorney about filing a medical malpractice lawsuit. We get battered on the witness stand by card sharks who intimate to the jury that I am a booze hound and I should have known about the risks of surgery, or just walking into a hospital at all. We lose the lawsuit, despite the surgeon himself not being able to explain how I supposedly lost my pancreas to gangrene before the hospital infection set in and he just "forgot" to notify us or any living person on the planet that I was out a major organ for a month.

It may have been the hurt I felt over the personal attacks that drove me to it, not the world going down in flames from chemicals and noxious food poisoning us all, pharmaceutical companies profiting obscenely from suffering diabetics, hospitals maiming or killing us when we ended up in their care or insurance lawyers waiting and ready to protect the hospitals from responsibility – all good for the economy mind you. But I finally decided I needed to know the truth: Was I crazy?

So I set out to see, not just one, but two different psychiatrists, just to make sure the second opinion confirmed the first. At this point, we were scientific about our approach to everything, and still not 100 percent trustful of just one medical opinion on any issue, so a whole team of university professors would have been welcome.

I sat in the Virginia Beach psychiatrist's office and asked him outright, "Do you think I am crazy?"

"No, you are probably not crazy, Mr. Vaughan," he replied.

"How do you know for sure?" I asked.

"You probably wouldn't be asking the question if you were. It's a healthy question for all of us to ask ourselves on occasion," he reassured me.

"Can you find that out for certain, with some kind of test or something?" I asked, as I had already prepared to request testing for myself.

"Sure. There are a few written tests I can administer that will gauge your overall mental health status and we can have a few evaluation sessions," he seemed delighted.

Both sets of tests, from both doctors, showed what I wasn't sure of: I wasn't insane. The last doctor I visited took in my history, recent and past, and offered to help me feel better about what I had lived through and what I was going to continue to go through for the rest of my life: the daily managing of a body kept alive through machines and medicine on the surface, but really, by the love I had for Shirley and our family beneath it and under the strain of it all. My family was worth it. My life was worth it. It was all worth one more day.

I wasn't crazy, but I was depressed. The depression was probably inevitable as the link between diabetes and depression is well established. Even without the craziness of the years following the TP, the fallout from the beyond brittle diabetes alone was enough to send me over the tipping point.

Unfortunately, depression is something I could have seen coming if I had known about the relationship between it and diabetes. According to an evaluation of 20 studies over the past 10 years, the prevalence rate of diabetics with major depression is three to four times greater than in the general population. While depression affects maybe three or five percent of the population at any given time, the rate is between 15 and twenty percent in patients with diabetes, according to the American Diabetic Association.

"One plus one equals much more than two when you add diabetes and depression," says Patrick Lustman, PhD, professor of medical psychology in the department of psychiatry at

Washington University School of Medicine in St Louis. "Because of physiologic and behavioral interactions between diabetes and depression, each becomes more difficult to control, increasing the risks of cardiovascular disease, diabetic retinopathy causing blindness, neuropathy and other complications." [1]

So, I took the Zoloft and joined the skyrocketing population of almost one in 10 or 27 million Americans who also took antidepressants as modern coping tools for modern life. The number of Americans using antidepressants doubled in only a decade, from 1996 to 2006, according to the study of nearly 50,000 children and adults in the medical journal *Archives of General Psychiatry*. As with the stunning statistics on diabetes and cancer, once again, I was saddened by the amount of company I encountered on the road back to health. [2]

Eventually, the tide turned and we noticed. We left the buggy apartment and returned to our family home, with the boxwood maze and the lady slipper orchid that was showing up regularly in the spring. We gratefully acknowledged to God that we had each other, and now, with our logs of concrete data and years of finding things out the hard way, we had a plan.

Succession planning and planting of a variety of vegetables meant something would be coming in most weeks of the summer as the spent plants were pulled out. This is also the best way to insure we were getting our monies' worth from our efforts. The amount of time and energy that is necessary to plan and grow your own food these days is worth the effort, especially as food prices continue to soar. As oil prices continue to go up, so will food prices, as most of our food is grown in an oil-dependent industrial agriculture system that trucks and ships food thousands of miles to market. A dime spent on seeds yields about one dollar's worth of produce. According to an *MSN Money* article, the five foods that are worth it to grow yourself are any high-producing vine vegetable, such as squash and cucumbers, peppers, lettuces, herbs and anything from a fruit tree. [1]

Joining the rest of the country's trendsetters on the hot pursuit of finding or growing the freshest local produce was a national food movement Shirley and I were now a part of – not as a fad for us, but as a life-saving measure for my body to insure we would have as many minutes and days together as possible. Apparently, a growing number of Americans were arriving at the same conclusions for their own health and economic reasons.

The largest U.S. seed company, W. Atlee Burpee & Co, reported selling twice as many seeds in 2008 as 2007, with half that increase from new customers. Seed Savers Exchange, a non-profit dedicated to preserving heirloom vegetables, sold 34,000 packets of seed in the first four months of 2008, exceeding total sales of 2007. [2] And in 2007, the Oxford American Dictionary voted the newly created word "locavore" – meaning people who buy and eat local food - as the word of the year. But the family gardening part of this trend, however novel it may have appeared to a new generation, wasn't new at all.

During World War II, when food rations and shortages became a way of life, commercially canned goods, fresh fruits and vegetables were scarce. To help ease the problem, the Department of Agriculture told Americans that if they wanted fresh fruits and vegetables, they would simply have to grow them for themselves. Thus the birth of the "Victory Garden," also referred to as a "Survivor Garden" was born. Within just two years, 1941 to 1943, 20 million Americans planted victory gardens and produced 40% of the country's food supply. [3]

As the summer wore on, we became more adventurous and decided we would like to take a trip to the ocean to find fresh shrimp and fish for the overflowing freezer. Shooting down winding country roads with the sun on our faces and the wind in our hair reminded us of a faraway time... a time when we didn't carry the locked briefcase with backup supplies of surgical steel lancets to mine my sore fingers for needed blood, hopefully-not-recalled test strips, an extra legally-allowed-to-be-20-percent-off-in-its-results glucometer, extra tubing for the insulin pump, needles for self injections if the pump fails, a nameless plastic bottle to dispose of needles so drug addicts wouldn't break into our home for fresh ones, extra enzymes and insulin labeled "human" but not really, a list of meds and doctors and cash for emergencies and glucose packets for low blood glucose levels - all considered drug paraphernalia that we could be arrested for transporting if we didn't keep it under lock and key in the bulky leather case.

Between the garden bursting with fresh food, our inspections of local farmers' markets and orchards, and trips to the ocean for fresh seafood, our life began to settle into a routine that revolved around all things nourishing, and peaceful. Our plan was simple. Our plan was, as always, peace. We wanted peaceful lives together. So much of our day to day existence was now dictated by tight schedules and chronicling of my every move… too much exercise, too little exercise, too many biscuits, not enough biscuits! We knew if we focused on the parts we had no control over, well, we knew where that would lead, and it wouldn't lead to peace.

The wonderful thing about a garden is, it will keep you engaged with life and what is real. And what is real is so magnificent, that we, all of us, really live off of the grace of God's goodness and our love for one another, whether we acknowledge this or not.

I'm not kidding about this backyard growing being a national trend by the time Shirley and I jumped on board. Not only had lots of people, I'll bet with health issues or trying to avoid them, read the regular news reports and studies linking processed food with chronic disease, but there were just as many people and institutions showing up with solutions to the problem and national question of "What Are We Going To Eat?" (see resources in back of book).

One group of people especially found success with returning to their roots for combating diabetes. Native American tribes from all parts of the country have experienced such high rates of Type 2 diabetes, in one *USA Today* article, a tribeswoman said it was the exception in her family if you didn't have diabetes. Thanks to national and local government-funded programs that focus on preserving and renewing cultural identity, Native Americans are successfully recovering from the epidemic.

"We've listened to tribe elders from the beginning, and through our Traditional Foods project, we've honored the concepts of harvesting, gathering and preparing traditional foods like squash and berries," says Dawn Satterfield, a team leader for the Native Diabetes Wellness Program at the CDC, that has worked with 17 tribal communities to improve access to local, fresh produce.[5]

From all outside appearances, Americans had determined that industrial systems of food growing and preparing might keep machinery humming, but it didn't keep people healthy. The national movement to remember how our grandparents grew wholesome food was a collective effort to ditch a system that didn't serve us, and instead, to serve ourselves heaping helpings of common sense and home-grown nourishment from our own backyards.

CHAPTER NINE:

Caring for the Caregiver, Shirley Shares Her Self-care Secrets

"Enjoy the little things, for one day you may look back and realize they were the big things."

—Robert Brault

How many lightning-bolt revelations did Dale Evans have with her feet in stirrups? I don't know, but I was on my gynecologist's table where I first realized I was probably overestimating my ability to have anything resembling my former life for myself in 2005, almost a year after Clyde lost his pancreas. After an hour of waiting in my doctor's plush lobby, flipping through women's magazines (you know, the ones showing you the life of manicures, pedicures and shopping sprees with girlfriends you should have) I was finally called back to the hot, small room for my annual exam.

As I passed by the fortressed window where the receptionist sat, I peeped in through the glass wall and discretely reminded her, "Remember, I told you I have to leave here by a certain time. My husband's life depends upon it! Don't let them keep me waiting much longer."

"Okay," she smiled reassuringly. And I believed her. So, in the small examination room, I stripped, pulled a blue paper almost impossible for me to find a few moments for myself. But over the past few years, I have found ways to keep my sanity and wellness, for both of our sakes. And let's face it; my self-care is just as important as my care for him. Without Shirley, there may be no Clyde. I have told my children that if I go first, I am willing him to one of them, but my goal is to outlive them all. I love my life, my children, my grandchildren and my husband. I am here for as long as God allows me to be, and continues to answer my prayers for patience and strength, and for that hoped-for day of peace.

How did I survive and handle taking on the role of researcher, dietician, nurse and constant companion? Through the four Ps: Prayer, Prevention, Pause, and my favorite, my own home-canned Peach Preserves in the spring and Plum preserves in the fall!

My first rule is prayer. Prayer for myself. It is like they say on an airplane; you must put on the oxygen mask for yourself before you can put the oxygen mask onto others. In my relationship with God, I always ask for patience, which helps me to pace myself. Well, there are two more Ps! As Clyde talked about in chapter three, that lady slipper orchid showing up in our yard the first spring after he lost his pancreas, and after our first year of learning how this was going to work, reminded me of my belief that God never promised us life would be fair, but He did promise to go through it with us every step of the way. I have looked for this saying on the internet, to see if someone said it first. I have not been able to find who said it first. There are all kinds of versions of it and it is so popular, I know I am not the only person living by its promise and wisdom.

My second rule is Prevention. An ounce of prevention is worth a pound of cure isn't just a saying, it is a wise fact penned by Benjamin Franklin — who was probably providing care for a sick person when he thought of it! Prevention includes following Clyde's diet for him and for me. One misstep during the day can result in both of us losing sleep all night with trying to raise or lower his blood glucose levels. And sleep is precious. Losing sleep for both of us means days of exhaustion until we are caught up on what we missed. So, walking the straight and narrow of prevention is a secret to keeping my sanity.

Along the road of prevention has been a lot of sacrifice. Some of what we've given up might seem small, but when you're the one doing the sacrificing, the loss can be heartbreaking. One of the hardest things, of the many, that we have given up has to be eating out at restaurants. We both enjoyed traveling up and down the East Coast in years past, and can give you a list of the best places to eat if you wanted one. One of our favorite places was in Pennsylvania in the Amish country. Clyde and I used to drive to Pennsylvania often for Japanese toy collector conventions. We knew the route to take through the back country to go by our favorite hideaways and still end up where we were going on time.

But restaurants these days are minefields for people with autoimmune disorders. Because menu items are rarely labeled with ingredients, like corn syrup and dextrose, to order blindly is a gamble we cannot afford to take anymore. Even helpful guides, like the *Fast Food Diabetes Pocket Guide*, can tell you what they think you can expect, but those guesstimates are not worth the risk for Clyde and I, and we unfortunately found this out the hard way, as it isn't just restaurant menus that are gambles on ingredients, but products in stores that change their ingredients without letting you know.

Like the rest of our journey through the loss of Clyde's pancreas, we found out that we have so much company on the road back to health, with so many people suffering from so many

- Add a recommended daily limit on added sugar consumption to the Nutrition Facts label,

- Make the Nutrition Facts label easier to understand, and

- Standard nutritional health symbols that appear on the fronts of food packages.

- List the percentages of key ingredients,

- List ingredients in an easy-to-read font and format, as displayed below. (Currently allowed label on left and proposed label on right, from their website, http://cspinet.org/foodlabeling/)

The CSPI's website points out the savings these sorts of no-brainer prevention tactics would have for society. "Modernization of nutrition and health information on food labels is an essential weapon in the fight against obesity and diet-related diseases. Cost-benefit analyses of previous food labeling reforms show that the cost of changing food labels is greatly outweighed by the health benefits of providing consumers with better label information." Of course, the ultimate prevention, as we found, is to grow it and can it yourself, eliminating the need or mystery of labels.

Another Prevention tactic is the travel case I have prepared for us; even visiting our children who live locally means being prepared for all scenarios with Clyde's health. The travel kit that I created and carry is in a brief case, and the reason for this is that in Virginia all medical syringes must be kept under lock and key for transporting them, otherwise an officer pulling you over for a busted tail light could end up charging you with transporting drug paraphernalia. Thank goodness I did not have to find THIS piece of information out the hard way!

And yes I did remake and keep that annual exam with my gynecologist, and all of my own preventive care doctor appointments.

My third rule is to Pause. I take thirty minutes a day to myself, no matter what. Sometimes, that thirty minutes is fifteen minutes in the morning and fifteen at night, or five minutes stolen here and there. In that precious thirty minutes what I need most is to just have my own thoughts.

My fourth rule is Peach Preserves in the spring and Plum Preserves in the fall, my own homemade kind, or something equally energy boosting! Because I am in charge of researching, planning and preparing Clyde's meals, I do eat healthier than most people. But because I do have a pancreas and am not diabetic, I do allow myself my "energy foods".

One of my favorite energy foods is the peach preserves I make from the peaches I freeze from spring harvests at plentiful local farms here in southeastern Virginia. In the fall, the plums are ripe and ready for picking and preserving. I make preserves like I make everything, taste tested as I go. I also make grape jelly from our grape vines. Again, all of this, picking and washing and then making the preserves and jellies does not have to be done at the same time. In fact, if you are like me, you don't have a whole day for this production. But fruit freezes well and will keep until you are ready to schedule a few hours to turn your kitchen into preserves production line.

Clyde does not get to be a taste tester of preserves because of the amount of sugar in them: one pound of sugar to one pound of fruit. Now you understand why this is an energy source! But these sorts of energy sources are to be used sparingly, as unused energy converts to fat in about two to four hours if it is not used. Clyde and I can both still fit into our wedding clothes, and we are determined to keep it that way!

What wisdom came to Dale Evans with her feet in real stirrups? As it turns out, Dale Evans suffered from diabetes for 36 years before talking about her condition publicly. In her first admission of her disease in an interview in *Diabetes Forecast* in March 2000, Evans said it was the insulin injections that prompted her to go public.

An actress, singer, an entertainer, and a best-selling author, she was married four times. Her marriage to the "king of the cowboys," Roy Rogers, lasted almost 51 years, until his death of congestive heart failure in 1998 at the age of 86. She wrote their theme song "Happy Trails."

Dale Evan's famous quote about suffering with diabetes is, "Life is not over because you have diabetes. Make the most of what you have, be grateful." [2] Our life was certainly not over when Clyde lost his pancreas and became a beyond brittle diabetic, but our life the way we knew it was. Who could have guessed forty years ago, when we said "in sickness and in health" that such a test of those wedding vows was on its way? Who knew our love for each other would help us survive the test? Well, maybe we did.

SHIRLEY'S PEACH PRESERVES

If you are pressed for time when the harvest comes in, buy the peaches anyway and freeze them. During the winter and early spring, I can usually find more time to make my preserves. This recipe is good, not only for peaches, but for all fruit preserves. I would share with you my homemade biscuit recipe – that is a great, almost necessary partner for the preserves – but I don't have a biscuit recipe. I just shake flour in a bowl and pour water in until it is the right consistency, make balls and bake. You can experiment with flour and water, which is the best way, to make your own! For the peach preserves, you will need:

1 pound peaches, peeled and sliced

1 pound sugar (depends on the fruit how sweet it is)

DIRECTIONS: Coat peaches with sugar, and let stand for 12 hours. Bring mixture slowly to a boil. Stir frequently. Boil gently until the fruit becomes clear and the syrup   drops bead by bead on a spoon. Let stand until cold. Skim off foam. Pack into jars and seal. Put jars in a hot water bath and boil about five minutes. Let jars stand until seal, after they are seal, let sit overnight to make sure all jars are sealed.

CHAPTER TEN:

Living Without A Pancreas

"It is not given to us to know which acts or by whom, will cause the critical mass to tip toward an enduring good. What's needed for dramatic change is an accumulation of acts, adding, adding to, adding more, continuing. We know that it does not take 'everyone on Earth' to bring justice and peace, but only a small, determined group who will not give up during the first, second, or hundredth gale."

— Clarissa Pinkola Estes

For the first time in nearly six years, Shirley and I sat in our family home in spring 2010 and just stared at each other. Was it true? Was the ride over? Did we really make it through the medical experiment of learning to live without my pancreas, solving a chemically-induced mystery illness, fighting a nepotistic town council, banishing an Agent Orange cloud from our neighborhood, losing a lawsuit to a last century cow dispute, being ostracized from our church for citizen activism/trouble-making, all while living nomadically in infested newlywed apartments and toting drug paraphernalia in locked luggage to avoid arrest?

Sitting in our family den beneath the painting of my father and brothers picking peanuts on the pine knot paneled wall with our spring garden visible through the glass back door, a question that had long awaited a calm moment to emerge finally did... could it be true that I was the only person who had "figured it out" for myself? (The living without the pancreas part, not the Agent Orange family cow feud parts.)

Even though the CDC and the National Centers for Health Statistics stated they did not have numbers on total pancreatectomies, TPs, because they were too rare to track, I still wondered if someone, *anyone* out there had survived losing their pancreas and was alive to tell about it. Even though I could have patrolled the garden paths for stray weeds with Sir Bentley all day, Shirley limited my intense workouts to two hours which left plenty of time to finally answer the question: was there anybody out there?

Right away, in a fairly quick internet search, the story of Betsy Hilfiger (the designer Tommy's sister), popped up. Ms. Hilfiger's story was featured on the Pancreas Center at Columbia University's website, who performed a prophylactic TP because she had tested positive for pre-cancerous cells in her pancreas. The story of Ms. Hilfiger popped up quickly, but contact information for her did not. [1]

In the same fashion as the children's story of *When You Give A Mouse A Cookie*, meaning, one thing leads to another, my search led me from one thought to another and one website to another until I amassed enough information on TPs to embolden me to start calling university centers individually to see if they would share their statistics or resources.

Every media officer I talked with was helpful, and even promised to look into my questions on TPs, but none of them, even the ones that called back days later, had any information for me. It was the media officer with Johns Hopkins that was the most helpful. She pointed me to the Johns Hopkins' online message board where I posted a request for information on TPs and survivors. A few weeks later, someone replied and told me about a small, self-run support group on a Yahoogroups' discussion board. The board listed around 70 members, but only around a dozen were active posters with six to 50 messages a month.

The group members were happy to share their stories of why they had TPs and how they were doing now. Some of the group members took part in groundbreaking surgical techniques, with the Da Vinci robot, or with the early detection offered by the National Familial Tumor Registry and CAPS, Cancer of the Pancreas Screening programs. While everyone's path to TP surgery was different, our shared experiences were revealed in a poll we conducted. One of the questions we asked was, Do you feel you had enough guidance on how to live without a pancreas? The overwhelming answer was no: minimal or no medical preparation and guidance after a TP equaled years of horrific stress on our bodies and families until everyone "figured it out" for themselves.

In an interview, Ted Levy, the Yahoogroup moderator, shared that even though his TP and follow-up were with Johns Hopkins, "the crème de la crème of medical care", he was not pre-pared for the aftermath of a TP.

"Everyone in the group survey said they did not get enough information to handle the diabetes, I will say no as well, despite being treated at Johns Hopkins and being surrounded by the best resources in the country or the world. Even though I have great medical care and my doctors are great. Even though it is a group of endocrinologists, they have very little experience with someone who has had a TP. Their experience is usually with people who are dying. That is why our Yahoogroup is for post-TP-diabetics, because everyone has the experience of losing the pancreas and becoming brittle diabetics," said Levy.

Another shared experience of the group was constantly correcting *doctors* who told them, during their aftercare, that they couldn't live without a pancreas. Jonathan Lightman, a lobbyist from California, said he grew so tired of correcting doctors that he began to quip, "Oh, did I say I had my pancreas removed? I meant to say I had pancakes for breakfast."

"My wife, Janice, and I both believe you have to be brilliant to survive the recovery from a TP, to figure it all out for yourself," shared Jonathan. If Jonathan is right, then the real tragedy is the one that will never be told. With no tracking of this rare surgery, how would we ever know who wasn't brilliant enough or supported enough, in my case, to "figure it out" in time?

While most group members agreed that they were not prepared for the difficult recovery from a TP and the inevitable beyond brittle diabetes, the path coming into a TP was different for everyone. And how you came into having a TP in the first place, sometimes determined how well you eventually did on the other side.

Liz, whose husband was the TP survivor, observed, "If you came into your TP through pancreatitis, you are probably still in pain and wondering if the surgery was the right thing to do. If you came into your TP through cancer, you are just grateful to be alive."

Of the various ways a patient can end up with a recommendation for a TP, the two main avenues were diseases of the pancreas, like the painful pancreatits, or the deadly but often symptomless pancreatic cancer.

Pancreatic cancer, a silent killer with few symptoms, claims the lives of 96 percent of its victims — most within a year of diagnosis. Even though it is only the 11th most common cancer in the United States, it is the fourth-leading cause of cancer death, because nearly all the patients die. Every year about 42,470 individuals are diagnosed and 35,240 a year die from the disease, according to the National Cancer Center with the National Institutes of Health (visit them at www.cancer.gov). The prognosis for pancreatic cancer is poor, as less than five percent are still alive five years after diagnosis and complete remission is rare.

The good news for cancer patients is that, "Any cancer can be cured if it's caught early enough," states leading Johns Hopkins cancer expert Dr. Bert Vogelstein, "Cancer develops in a place in the body, in an organ. As long as it hasn't spread to other organs, it generally can be removed."

In an interview in July 2010 in *Johns Hopkins* magazine, Vogelstein states in the last 25 years, he has seen cancer go from a "black box" that medical science did not understand to a "revolution" in detection and treatment. In fact was Vogelstein's seminal discoveries that helped establish cancer as a genetic disease.

Unfortunately, as the article points out, "heredity accounts for just five percent of all malignancies. The other 95 percent happen because cells sometimes make mistakes when they copy their DNA. These mistakes are exacerbated by exposure to such things as cigarette smoke, ultraviolet light, toxins, and infections."[2] Not surprisingly, the article echoes the findings of the US President's Council on Cancer in 2010, our toxic food and environment can alter our bodies at the cellular level and trigger cancer to form and thrive on those same toxins. [3]

As the *Johns Hopkins* article, "Detecting A Cure" writes, the real challenge for pancreatic cancer patients has been the early detection of the usually silent disease. "Existing tests such as pap smears for cervical cancer and mammograms for breast cancer are a testament to the effectiveness of early detection; they have significantly reduced deaths caused by these cancers. But even these tests aren't perfect. They depend on the skill of the lab technician and the capability of the imaging, which means some cancers go missed. They also result in many false positives, which cause unnecessary anxiety for patients and can lead to unnecessary invasive procedures, such as biopsies, which carry the risk of complications and even death.

"This is where the new generation of diagnostic tests comes into play. Doctors will be able to detect many cancers through new tests based on molecular 'biomarkers' such as gene mutations or increases in proteins that definitively indicate a certain cancer."

The same *John Hopkins* article features Levy's story of catching his cancer in time with a combination of identifying at-risk genetic groups and families and early detection testing and scans. In 1982, Levy's father died of pancreatic cancer, and his uncle died of it four years before. When a close friend became ill with the disease in 2001, Levy's wife began an internet search to help her friend, and stumbled on a link for the National Familial Pancreas Tumor Registry at Johns Hopkins Hospital. Through the registry, Levy was contact by and began participating in the CAPS program, Cancer of the Pancreas Screening study. The study screens people with a high familial risk for pancreatic cancer through an aggressive program using advanced imaging. The geneticist recommended that Levy also be tested for mutations in the BRCA genes, which were originally associated with breast cancer and now are also associated with pancreatic cancer. As an Ashkenazi Jew (of Eastern European descent), Levy was much more likely to have this mutation. During follow up tests in January 2004, his doctor concluded that a detected lesion was intraductal papillary mucinous neoplasm, IPMN, or precancerous cells — and that it appeared to be progressing. In the meantime, another warning sign had come in: the results of Levy's genetic tests. He had a BRCA2 mutation. IPMNs are thought inevitably to become invasive cancer — and the lesion was already at one centimeter. Levy remembered his uncle and father, and made his decision.

The article continues, "The tests they are working on will help best decide who needs surgery and who does not." [4]

"By dying from pancreatic cancer my father saved my life," Levy shared with me. "Had that not happened, I wouldn't have been in an early detection program. Once I found out, the rest of my family members were tested, including my children and my sister's children, and two of them were positive. Everyone is being followed aggressively."

As medical science becomes more and more adept at helping pancreatic cancer patients become survivors, and identifying their family members for risks, it seems inevitable that TPs will become more common - and Levy's Yahoogroups' role in providing support and information for new post-TP/ beyond brittle diabetics more crucial for their recovery.

Another Yahoogroup member, Annamarie Ibrahim, from Green Valley, California, has 30 family members participating in the registry and study through the Mayo Clinic. Seven members of Annamarie's family have died from pancreatic cancer. Annamarie underwent a TP in September 2007 due to the detection of an IPMN.

"After a year of pancreatitis, just prior to my surgery for IPMN, we went to a Diabetes Pump Users Group. I quickly discovered that there is diabetes and then there is DIABETES. Did it scare me? Yes, but not nearly as much as remembering the challenges my other family members faced without a positive outlook from their diagnosis. TP wasn't an option for my other family members because it was too late," writes Annamarie in an email. "My husband and I looked at each other and it wasn't even necessary to decide if I was going to have the surgery or not....It was a no brainer!"

Lightman says the difference between his support pre- and then post-surgery could not have been more disparate. "This was ridiculously harsh, *ridiculously harsh*. When I came home the hardest thing was eating and learning how to digest. Every time I ate I felt like I had the worst jet lag in the world, times a factor of 20. I was freezing. My brain didn't understand what was going on," said Lightman, told me. "The medical community said the first year would be tough, but when I was complaining after two years, they said that didn't make sense, why didn't you tell us about this earlier? I said, 'I did'. They tried to blame me but I was talking to them the whole time.

"In my experience, there is no real game plan in the after plan for the TP. Going into the surgery everyone was phenomenal. I had meetings with everyone before, but afterwards, nothing. I felt extremely frustrated. I have figured it out on my own and through the list servs (Yahoogroup) and through trial and error. That is basically what it has been. One thing I can say is there is no way to get back to normal, that road doesn't even exist. It is all about reframing. I have chronic management of chronic pain and that is separate and aside from the fact that the cancer might come back."

Lightman says he has given a lot of thought to why recovery from a TP is so difficult and guidance so rare. "I think in our culture, unless it is something we can visibly see, you think when you have a surgery, you get better. That is not the case here. You have this surgery and your life becomes about management. With me, I am in incredible, chronic discomfort. My kidneys and other organs have migrated to these empty spaces and are causing me pain. People are alive, but in a very, very altered state. And of course everybody is an individual, but I think the common thread that everybody feels is very isolated. What is hard for me is that no one has exactly the same issues. It is hard enough dealing with this by myself. When people would post their phone numbers on the Yahoogroup, I would call them instead of trying to connect online."

Lightman said it was his reframing techniques and drive to understand what was happening to him that helped him to cope with daily living. "Reframing for me means not focusing on what am I not able to do, but what can I do. For example, when I was in the hospital for the surgery, for ten days, with all these tubes coming out of me - my eyesight was so messed up, I couldn't see to read - but I decided that I was going to figure out what was in my control. I decided that if the only two things in my control were brushing my teeth and shaving, then I would have the whitest teeth and closest shave of anyone in that hospital.

"Now, I am often looking like I am having a bad day, and people ask me, 'Oh are you having a bad day?' And if I were to answer honestly, I would say, no every minute of every day is a bad day. So, I have to reframe by asking what I can do."

Even though some Yahoogroup members were active posters in the online discussion, some, who wanted to remain anonymous, sent us these kinds of messages:

"I am one of the few who suffered multiple, severe and life-threatening complications from my TP/ICT. It has made my life worse than ever expected. I'm often reluctant to share on the message board because for most this surgery is an answer to prayers."

And then there were TP survivors, like Loma, who not only survived their TP and beyond brittle aftermath, they resumed their fairly normal lives, eventually. For the opposite reason from the above member, Loma also said she rarely posted on the

Yahoogroup because she was doing so well, she didn't want to discourage others who were suffering. "I read so many stories about bad things since surgeries, I guess I am an oddity," she told me.

Loma is a retired oncology nurse in Indiana who had her pancreas, spleen and gallbladder removed on May 7, 2003, when an emergency surgery for pain turned out to be cancer. "All my cancer was contained in the duct so I did not have to have chemo treatments. I have thought many times about writing a book on how I was a nurse working at the cancer center administering chemo to patients and then I became a cancer patient," she said.

"The surgery made me diabetic instantly. I knew nothing about what to do. I think this is where they dropped the ball at the hospital. I came home with nothing, no information, other than I was going to have to take enzymes the rest of my life. I did not go on an insulin pump for a few months. I was in the hospital eight days and then when I came home there was a home care nurse that came and checked on me, my dressing and incision. But that was it. I am lucky to have a husband who is wonderful and looked after me."

Because her TP was seven years ago, Loma says she has seen the number of people who have had TPs increase on the Yahoogroup. "There were fewer of us a few years ago than there are now. At least who are on the internet and talking about how awful they are doing. It is a miracle that I did so well and I feel that I need to be able to do something to help these people. I would have given anything if I had had ME to tell me what to do with this pump in the beginning. Even though I am doing well now, there are still some things that are going to be the same with what we all went through to figure out how to help ourselves."

Loma feels she is lucky because two weeks after the TP she was able to walk a few miles for exercise, and within six weeks she was playing golf again. "I was 60 when I had my surgery and I was in good health. I was swinging a golf club six weeks after I had my surgery. The way my incision went, it went with my swing," said Loma. "I had grandkids and a life to live and I decided to beat this thing."

Like most of the group members, Loma said one of her biggest hurdles post-TP was gaining and keeping enough weight on a body that food just passes right through, even with pharmaceutical grade enzymes to help. In listening to everyone compare notes on trying to put weight on after the surgery, I remembered my own doctor warning me when he was discharging me in Norfolk that I could expect to be the skeletal 128 pounds I was then for the rest of my life. I told him then to let me get home to my wife and her cooking and we would see about that. I was right. Shirley's Southern cooking did plump me back up to my former normal weight of 162 pounds. I wonder if she cooked for the group members for a month-long TP retreat in our backyard if she could fatten-up some of them? I know she would give it her best effort if given the chance.

The food issue, what to eat and which enzymes to take, was another shared experience with the group members. As Loma, who was doing great but still struggled with a diet plan, shared, "This is a constant and ongoing trial on what I can eat and what I can't eat. There are some things I can't eat because of the way I am re-plumbed after the surgery. Not everything digests the way it used to either. Finding somebody who will tell me what kind of diet I am supposed to be on or what kind of enzymes to take has been impossible. My endocrinologist at Indiana University doesn't know, and if he doesn't, who does? A lot of this I have had to learn on my own. But, I can also eat something today and then two weeks from now it doesn't agree with me at all. Maybe what I eat won't affect me for days, because it takes longer to affect me."

Loma, along with many other group members, feels frustrated by her desire to help others. "Why did I get so lucky? I don't know. I feel so bad for so many of these patients who hardly have a life. After all these years, that there has been nothing to help these people is awful. I wish there was something I could do."

The question at the back of my mind that needed a quiet moment in our lives to emerge, and finally did in 2010, found the answer was, no, I am not alone. I was torn between feeling grateful for the company and devastated that so many of us existed. As more information on what IS known about pancreatic surgeries and their aftermath surged through the portal of my home computer, so did more questions, like, is there currently a more accepted way to treat an ailing pancreas?

It was the media officer for Johns Hopkins, who pointed us to their message boards, who also offered to educate us on the Whipple, a surgical procedure on the head of the pancreas perfected and performed at John Hopkins. [5]

The Whipple procedure, also called a pancreaticoduodenectomy, is generally the removal of the gallbladder, common bile duct, part of the duodenum, and the head of the pancreas, according to the Sol Goldman Pancreatic Cancer Research Center at John Hopkins. After removal of these structures the remaining pancreas, bile duct and the intestine is sutured back into the intestine to direct the gastrointestinal secretions back into the gut.

Also called a pancreatic resection, the Whipple was first described in the 1930's by Allan O. Whipple, MD, of New York Memorial Hospital (now called Memorial Sloan-Kettering). Forty years after its creation, in the 1970's, the mortality rate for the Whipple operation was very high. Up to 25 percent of patients died from the surgery, states the Center for Pancreatic and Biliary Diseases at the University of Southern California, USC. [6]

"This experience of the 1970's is still remembered by some physicians who are reluctant to recommend the Whipple operation," states the USC website. "Today the Whipple operation has become an extremely safe operation in the USA. At tertiary care centers where a large numbers of these procedures are performed by a selected few surgeons, the mortality rate from the operation is less than four percent. Studies have shown that for good outcomes from the Whipple surgery, the experience of the center and the surgeon is important."

The most striking information we found on pancreas surgery reinforced our belief that the loss of my pancreas, through a risky and unnecessary intubation of the head of the pancreas that led to an infection, should never have happened. Surgeons and hospitals who have been "practicing" performing the revered Whipple operation since 1930, now say they are safe only if performed by an experience surgeon at a university center specializing in pancreatic surgeries.

"Recent studies from Johns Hopkins and Memorial Sloan Kettering have shown that outcome from surgery for a Whipple operation is dependent on the experience of the hospital and the surgeon performing the surgical operation…

"The American Cancer Society recommends that the Whipple operation should be performed in a center that is experienced and does high volume of these complex surgical procedures to ensure the best outcome," states the USC website.

The overall survival rate of the Whipple operation is about 20 percent at five years after surgery. Patients without the spread of cancer into their lymph nodes may have up to a 40 percent survival rate. For patients with low grade or benign cancers, the operation is usually curative, states USC.

Patients who had Whipple procedures did not necessarily become diabetic afterward. Because only the head of the pancreas was removed, pancreatic tissue remained. "Our experience has been that patients who are diabetic at the time of surgery or who have an abnormal blood sugar level that is controlled on a diet prior to surgery have a high chance for the severity of the diabetes becoming worse after the surgery. On the other hand patients who have completely normal blood sugar prior to surgery with no history of diabetes and do not have chronic pancreatitis have a low probability of developing diabetes after the Whipple operation," states USC.

Translation: Unlike a TP, a Whipple operation may not leave the patient a beyond brittle diabetic facing a "figure it out for yourself" scenario. The biggest complication post-Whipple is that in 25 percent of surgeries the stomach may remain paralyzed for up to four to six weeks and the patient will need to be fed through a feeding tube.

We wondered, at some point in our wonderings, if the infection in my pancreas from the hospital germ had been caught in time, and I could get to a qualified hospital, and monkeys could, well, never mind… would I have been a candidate for a pancreas transplant? According to Cedars-Sinai, the answer is no. In 2009, *U.S. News & World Report* Best Hospitals issue, Cedars-Sinai ranked among America's best hospitals in kidney disease. They are also one of a select few medical centers in Southern California performing kidney-pancreas transplants, so they know what they are talking about. And according to their website, "pancreas transplantation is used to prevent or reverse secondary complications of diabetes. The treatment is reserved for patients who are undergoing kidney transplantation and are also Type 1 diabetic. Diabetic patients who have already undergone kidney transplantation are also candidates. The procedure is restricted to this patient population because pancreas transplantation alone is not a lifesaving procedure." [7]

Who else might be considered and pitched the option of a TP? If the Yahoogroup members are a representative sampling of TP survivors, and it appears they are the only sample official or unofficial in the world, then the 80,000 Americans a year affected by pancreatitis could be lining-up for the surgery, or a version of it.

Chronic pancreatitis, an inflammation or scarring of the pancreas, is a life-threatening condition that destroys the pancreas and often results in severe abdominal pain, weight loss, fever, nausea, vomiting and, in some cases, cancer. Because of a fairly new, pioneering treatment to transplant the patients' own insulin-producing islet cells into their liver, pancreatitis sufferers have a better chance of avoiding the beyond brittle aftermath of a TP only. The TP/ICT, islet cell transplantation, is not an option for pancreatic cancer patients, as the possibility of transplanting precancerous cells into the liver is too dangerous.

In a TP/ICT, after removing the pancreas, physicians prepare the gland in the hospital's lab, while the patient waits in surgery, and isolate the insulin-producing cells of the pancreas. The islet cells are then taken back to the operating room, where they are injected through a catheter into a vein in the patient's liver. By transplanting the patient's own islets cells, there is no risk of rejection as in other organ transplants, and the cells lodge in the liver and make insulin.

While ICT is successful today, the transplanting of islet cells to "cure" diabetes predates the 1922 invention of purified insulin for human injection. "The first report of primitive islet transplantation as a treatment for diabetes was in 1894; Dr Watson Williams and Mr Harsant in Bristol (U.K.) transplanted portions of a sheep pancreas subcutaneously into a 15-year-old boy suffering from diabetic ketoacidosis. This was well before our current understanding of xenorejection; this graft was quickly rejected in this non-immunosuppressed patient," states a 2006 article in the magazine *Clinical Science*.[8]

Even though the point of transplanting the insulin producing cells in the liver is to avoid severe diabetes, ICT does not guarantee the patient will *not* become diabetic. As the Schulze Diabetes Institute at the University of Minnesota says, if the patient wants to trade chronic pancreatitis pain for the possibility of severe diabetes, this is now an option. "The probability of islet success is highest in those individuals who have had no previous direct surgery on the body and tail of the pancreas (such as a Puestow or Whipple procedure). For relief from the debilitating pain of chronic pancreatitis, patients have to accept the possibility of diabetes. If diabetes is prevented, it is a bonus."[9]

It was the Yahoogroup members who had opted for TP or TP/ICT due to pancreatitis that expressed the most disappointment, and even anger, over their or their spouse's surgery, usually because the pain of pancreatitis that prompted the surgery did not improve or only slightly improved. One member said she would not recommend a TP to anyone unless they had the islet cell transplant with the surgery to prevent the shock of severe and lifelong diabetes, and that she was doing well post-TP/ICT.

Another new Yahoogroup member posted to ask for help following a TP for chronic pancreatitis, CP, illustrated the possibility of ongoing pain post-TP:

"Hi. I am new to this group. I had my TP surgery on 7/9/09, after years of CP and constant pain. In the year (almost) since this surgery, my health and quality of life is not nearly as well as it was before the surgery. My doctors basically suggested the pancreas be removed due to constant pain; already had a portion of the pancreas and spleen removed a few years ago; and the fact that my ducts were very twisted and shriveled that they could not get an ERCP scope through them. My pancreas surgeon did advise me that having this surgery would not guarantee that I would be pain free, and he was right. I still have the same 'pancreatitis type' pain as I've had all along, and still require the use of strong narcotics (I'm on the fentanyl patch and percocet 3 times a day. I had this surgery done In the hopes of getting off the narcotics.

"Has anyone else had this problem? I do not understand how I could still have the constant pancreatitis pain with no pancreas? Any feedback would help."

One seasoned member's response was a formula for taking pharmaceuticals to avoid a "trail-off" effect of painkillers and to find an authentic acupuncturist for pain management.

Another Yahoogroup member posted: "My wife had a TP/ICT back in June 09. This surgery was not the end of her nightmares but only the beginning. For anyone thinking about this surgery you better do your homework. I think the questions you need to be looking at are how many people undergoing this surgery actually return to work.......along with how many have improved overall health after the surgery! Personally I would not undergo this surgery unless my options were choosing between the surgery and suicide because the chronic pancreatitis is so bad! Has anyone suffering from pancreas disease had any success with a celiac block or pain pump? My wife's medical bills are closing in on the $400,000 mark and her monthly meds run $3,000 per month. Be careful what you wish for!"

While I felt at times like a living medical experiment over these past years, Daniel O'Brien, also a group member, really was, as his TP/ICT surgery was the first in the world with a robot for a surgeon. The advantage of the Da Vinci robot for the pancreas removal allowed the surgeons to preserve and leave intact the spleen.

"My TP/ICT was different. I was the first attempted in the world 'full pancreatectomy/islet cell transplant' that was attempted with the Da Vinci surgical robot, which failed during surgery and has really messed up my insides. I didn't have it done conventionally. They do distal pancreatectomies with it, but mine was the first 'full' and second when done with the ICT. They did the first one distal, about six months before mine. You can read about THAT one here:

http://www.sciencedaily.com/releases/2007/05/070531204139.htm

"Same doctors, same hospital, different results. The robot ceased to function during surgery and the surgeon had to convert to conventional but the damage was done," wrote Daniel in an email.

While apparently many, but not most, of us beyond brittle TP survivors and our families suffered shock and a lack of knowledge of how to care for ourselves in those first months and years after a TP - and some of us were still suffering years later - the truth of the future of TP was experienced by Lightman in what he calls, an "epiphany" at a formal dinner in Washington, DC in 2007.

Jonathan's success with reframing helped to empower himself to become an activist for pancreatic cancer research, which lead to the moment of his epiphany.

"After the first year, I really wanted to do things. When you are laid up, all of a sudden you feel like you can't contribute. Well, I am a professional lobbyist, and that is what I decided to do.

Within the California state legislature, I got a senator to sponsor a bill and go on record to increase funding for pancreatic cancer. I threw parties for the Pancreatic Cancer Action Network. We had Jeopardy game. I heard Betsy Hillfiger speak in Beverly Hills this past November," said Lightman.

In 2007, Lightman flew from California to Washington, DC with a group of celebrities and supporters of the Pancreatic Cancer Action Network, PanCan, to petition the US Congress to fund research into early detection and treatment of pancreatic cancer. The celebrities included Cindy Landon, wife of *the Little House on the Prairie* television star, Michael Landon, who was of Jewish descent and who died from pancreatic cancer in 1991.

"In my 30 years of advocacy, the last 19 as a professional registered lobbyist, this was the most intensely personal lobbying effort in which I had ever participated," Lightman said.

Lightman said his epiphany came after a dinner during the DC trip featuring a speaker – a surgeon from Johns Hopkins - describe the current expectations for detection and treatment for pancreatic cancer. Lightman said he stood to ask the speaker a question about the reality of recovery from TP and ended up sharing his story of having his pancreas removed to avoid the fatal outcome of his IPMN diagnosis. Neither the surgeon nor the crowd had heard of such a possibility.

"After the dinner I was surrounded, engulfed, by hundreds of grieving families who wanted to know why their loved ones did not know to have the surgery I had. And that's when I had this epiphany. None of them would have cared if I were lying on the floor with spit coming out of my mouth. If I were their loved one, I would be alive and that is all they would care about," Lightman said.

And this is perhaps, the epiphany we all share. No matter what sort of hell we faced in our recovery from the TP, one more day with the people we loved and who loved us, and whose lives were going to be forever altered by grief if we gave up too soon, was worth it. This is what matters most to us, the love we share with our family and friends and the precious moments we have together, even when those moments are sleepless, anxious nights and frantic, desperate days. One more minute of one more day with them, was worth it all.

I began this book with Shirley and I riding the Jamestown ferry and contemplating a mid-river view of America's birthplace for a reason. Not only was this our favorite getaway, but the road trips through Jamestown and Williamsburg put us into the mind of survival and what was it like in the "olden day" and the gratitude we have for our "modern" lives. And we are grateful. But that doesn't mean that we aren't also wise and experienced enough to know that something has gone terribly wrong with our country due to its irrational dedication to the industrial ideals that landed on that beach at Jamestowne, a mere 400 years ago. We know, as many Americans are remembering, there were other ideals that landed there as well, ones that are attracting more attention in our current environment as the majority of Americans are reading health reports predicting what their lives are destined to look like as they age, if they already aren't burdened with the expense and debilitation of chronic illness directly attributed to medical mishap, chemical poisoning or the Standard American Diet, also known as SAD.

Living without a pancreas, and as a human guinea pig, forced me to think about the ongoing battle of those New World ideals in a way I had not considered before and may not have ever considered. It is amazing, and reassuring, how much company I find these days with so many people breaking free of compliant cog conditioning and instead, take charge of their lives, from simple acts like questioning labels to growing a portion of our own food.

What I believe, and have experienced firsthand, is that most of our modern systems – including medicine, chemicals and food production - are indeed, machinery, and if this machinery is going to serve us and our loved ones with integrity, instead of using us as cogs in its self-perpetuating machinery, then we, the possessors of hearts of courage and compassion and minds of common sense, will need to show up and inject into this machinery the necessary components to make it work for us, and not against us. This can be a tall order for us when we are already sick and suffering the human consequences from modern life's medical, chemical and agri-business systems. But the information on how consumers in a consumer-driven economy can take back their health and turn around the machinery already exists in that rabbit hole called the internet. All that is really left to us to do is to find the will to act. Fortunately, the inspiration for action is usually standing right beside us, in the form of the person, or people, who make our lives worth living. It is sort of an old-fashioned notion, love and dedication and commitment, but they are the foundation of those other old-fashioned ideals that landed at Jamestowne, the ideals of liberty and freedom and individual choice. And in the end, they are the only things that have ever served us or saved us.

AFTERTHOUGHTS...

A few of the Yahoogroup members generously agreed to share with the readers of this book the advice they wished they could have given to themselves in the beginning of their TP aftermath:

Jonathan shares: "Just because you make it through the surgery doesn't mean you are out of the woods. All of this is philosophically eye awakening experience. It is very weird because even though my life is so ridiculously complicated but I don't know that I would trade these past three years because I have seen the world through such a different lens. To see that really, really bad things can happen but that they are really good things, can happen when I try to approach the world from a place of what is my potential instead of what is my limit. But in retrospect, I would never have thoughts these things without this experience.

"You have to be super brilliant to be able to survive this sort of thing. This last hospital experience the nurses were convinced that I knew what I was doing and the nurses would ask simple questions but I would give them complicated answers and then they would need fifteen levels of approval to get anything done and then they finally said, 'Okay, we'll let you do whatever you want.' You can do your own research and you can be brave and brilliant enough to really be in charge of your own health."

Annamarie shares: "S-L-O-W D-O-W-N.....You'll need to become very 'in-tune' with your body and you'll discover things about yourself that you never thought possible. If you're going too fast, you'll never learn the lesson and you'll crash...literally, and you'll be forced to learn the hard way. Will reading my post stop you from doing things you're not supposed to? No, that's a guarantee. But, as you go through each rough experience and each joyful one...take a moment to learn and then take two moments to share your insights with someone else.

"Number one..... stay away from negative and uneducated people. Especially when they are wearing medical clothing. Staying positive is a choice. Yes, I have my days....some of them are especially rough. BUT, don't just pull yourself back up...PUSH AS HARD AS YOU CAN and ASK OTHERS FOR HELP. Learn to laugh at the 'unique' situations where you will find yourself. This is a joke that only this group will understand but...carry air freshener. Your gas will be worse than the dog's and you can't blame it on them because even the dog will run away."

Liz shares: "I would like to add to your observations of the value of a support system in the recovery from this surgery. I am convinced that our six children have contributed enormously to my husband's recovery and positive mindset. They took turns keeping me company at the hospital, brought our grandchildren to visit, we all celebrated father's day together. The hospital had never seen such a visiting crowd, just as well that there was a patio where we could all enjoy each .other's company. The IV pole was one of the 'guests'. After discharge our family developed a schedule so that we both had support. It is not quite three months post-Whipple, and my husband was readmitted for complications, probably due to the formation of some clots, so he is being cautiously optimistic about the prognosis."

William shares: "Kim and I will be happy to share Kim's TP/ICT experience with others. I agree with what Liz is saying. Do not consider pancreas surgery unless you have a very good at home support group. At the very least you will need one medical advocate that goes with you on Doctor and Testing appointments. Kim has had over 140 of these types of visits since Jan 2008. She takes 40 pills per day and takes an average of two insulin units four times per day. Kim uses a special alarm clock that can be scheduled to go off every hour to remind her of medicine times. Be happy!"

The information offered in this book doesn't stop here! Please take time to go through the rich resources and options for support offered in the following pages. There are also tips on blood glucose control and enzyme dosing, as well as my diet plan and citations for every study or fact mentioned in this book!

RESOURCES AND SUPPORT

PATIENT EDUCATION AND ADVOCACY:
Did You Know?

The seventh annual HealthGrades Patient Safety in American Hospitals study, released in March 2010, painted a dire picture of patient safety in U.S. hospitals, especially those that ranked outside of the top five percent.

The study, which analyzed nearly 40 million hospitalization records, found that nearly one million patient-safety incidents occurred among Medicare patients from 2006-2008. Sick Care "Patient-Safety (error) incidents" are, in essence, medical mistakes that cause patients harm or, for one in 10, costs them their life.

The researchers noted major discrepancies between the top ranking hospitals and poorly performing ones, with those visiting the top five percent experiencing 43 percent fewer patient-safety incidents. If the lower ranking hospitals were brought up to this level, it's estimated that over 218,500 patient-safety incidents and 22,500 deaths could have been avoided, along with $2 billion saved.

When you seek treatment at a hospital for one particular medical problem, you don't expect to acquire an additional injury, infection, or other serious condition during your stay. Although some complications may be unavoidable, too often patients suffer from injuries or an illness that could have been prevented if the hospital adopted safe practices and developed better systems that support improved patient safety.

Patient safety is not a new issue. Hospitals have increasingly implemented strategies aimed at reducing preventable patient safety events over the past ten years since the Institute of Medicine published To Err is Human: Building a Safer Health System. This landmark report published in 1999 focused the nation's attention on patient safety.

While hospitals have made progress, medical mistakes still occur at an alarming rate. The incidence rate of medical harm occurring is estimated to be over 40,000 per day according to the Institute for Healthcare Improvement. In 2002, the Centers for Disease Control and Prevention estimated that all hospital-acquired infections were associated with 99,000 deaths per year. For example, The Joint Commission, a nonprofit agency that certifies health care organizations, reports that only 89% of the facilities surveyed in 2008 met the patient safety goal for following the Centers for Disease Control and Prevention's (CDC) hand hygiene guidelines for preventing the spread of infection.

The federal government is taking steps to make hospitals safer, encouraging hospitals to adopt safe practices by establishing a zero-tolerance policy for preventable hospital-acquired complications. As of October 2008, the Centers for Medicare and Medicaid Services (CMS) no longer reimburses hospitals for the care of hospital-acquired conditions (such as certain infections, advanced bed sores, or fractures) and preventable medical errors that should never happen, such as performing surgery

on the wrong body part.

These hospital-acquired conditions can be reasonably prevented through the use of evidence-based guidelines and hospitals are now required to indicate whether these conditions are present at the time of admission. This new reporting requirement has increased the focus on patient safety at hospitals and will enable further analysis when the Medicare 2009 data are available. *From the HealthGrades' Seventh Annual Patient Safety in American Hospitals Study.*

Find How Your Hospital or Doctor Ranks at the HealthGrades website. Or share your experience by ranking your hospital or doctor. www.healthgrades.com.

Books:

How to Survive Your Doctor's Care. Pamela Gallin.
Making Informed Medical Decisions: Where to Look and How to Use What You Find. Nancy Oster, Lucy Thomas, Darol Joseff, MD.
Working with Your Doctor: Getting the Healthcare You Deserve. Nancy Keene.

Websites and Organizations:

Find a Qualified Doctor or Hospital. American College of Surgeons. http://www.facs.org/patienteducation/patient-resources/surgery.html

The Center for Medical Consumers. The Center for Medical Consumers, a non-profit 501(C)3 advocacy organization, was founded in 1976 with this philosophy: Whenever long-term drug therapy, elective surgery, or any other major treatment is prescribed, the question of whether the treatment has been proven safe and effective should come up. And the prescribing physician should be expected to cite the relevant studies. We want people not only to ask such questions but to explore the answers they receive from their physicians. http://medicalconsumers.org/

Speak Up. Ten comprehensive, easy-to-read brochures written to help patients "speak up" to health professionals about their care to ensure that they receive safe, thorough medical attention. Topics include "How to Avoid Mistakes in Your Surgery," "Five Things That You Can Do To Prevent Infection," and "Know Your Rights." http://www.jointcommission.org/PatientSafety/SpeakUp/

Agency for Research Healthcare and Quality. This federal government website, under the US Department of Health and Human Services, includes clinical practice guidelines for both the physician and consumer. http://www.ahrq.gov/

Reports:

HealthGrades Seventh Annual Patient Safety in American Hospitals Study. www.healthgrades.com/media/DMS/pdf/Patient SafetyInAmericanHospitalsStudy2010.pdf

Extending the Cure. The Extending the Cure project is a research and consultative effort that frames the growing problem of anti-biotic resistance as a challenge in managing a shared societal resource. The inaugural report of Extending the Cure provides an objective evaluation of a number of policies to encourage patients, health care providers, and managed care organizations to make better use of existing antibiotics and to give pharmaceutical firms greater incentives to both develop new antibiotics and care about resistance to existing drugs. www.extendingthecure.org

Support Groups:

Total Pancreactomy Survivors Yahoogroup. This group is listed on the John Hopkins Sol Goldman Pancreatic Cancer Research

health problems due to exposure to the household toxins listed above, particularly worrisome are the effects that these toxins may have on babies growing in their mothers' wombs.

A study conducted in 2004 by the Environmental Working Group found that umbilical cord blood from 10 newborns contained chemicals used in consumer products, pesticides, and by-products from gasoline, garbage, and the burning of coal.

On average, the blood from each newborn contained 200 industrial pollutants and chemicals. Of the 287 toxins that were found in the newborns' blood, 180 are known to cause cancer in humans or animals, 217 are known to be toxic to the brain and nervous system, and 208 are known to cause birth defects or abnormal development in animal tests.

Books:

Slow Death by Rubber Duck: The Secret Dangers of Everyday Things, Pollution is no longer just about belching smokestacks and ugly sewer pipes—now, it's personal. The most dangerous pollution, it turns out, comes from commonplace items in our homes and workplaces. To prove this point, for one week authors Rick Smith and Bruce Lourie ingested and inhaled a host of things that surround all of us. Ultimately hopeful, the book empowers readers with some simple ideas for protecting themselves and their families, and changing things for the better.

ToolKits:

Burn Wise Kit. Environmental Protection Agency. Burn Wise is an educational campaign that encourages people to burn only dry, seasoned wood or wood pellets and includes messages about cost savings (i.e., burning less wood), improved safety and health benefits. Because being more energy efficient means burning less wood. http://www.epa.gov/burnwise/burnwisekit.html

Air Defenders, www.airdefenders.org, an educational tool kit for teachers.

Website and Organization Resources:

GAIA: Global Alliance for Incinerator Alternatives. GAIA is a worldwide alliance of more than 500 grassroots groups, non-governmental organizations, and individuals in over 80 countries whose ultimate vision is a just, toxic-free world without incineration. We work both *against* incinerators and *for* safe, sustainable and just alternatives. www.no-burn.org.

Ingredient Central is run by the American Cleaning Institute, the Consumer Specialty Products Association, and the Canadian Consumer Specialty Products Association who have developed an ingredient communication initiative as a way to provide consumers with information about the ingredients in products in four major categories: air care, automotive care, cleaning, and polishes and floor maintenance products. Lists of ingredients for most of the cleaning products consumers use every day are now available at their website: www.cleaninginstitute.org/ingredientcentral.

Environmental Working Group. The mission of the EWG is to use the power of public information to protect public health and the environment. EWG is a 501(c)(3) non-profit organization, founded in 1993. In 2002, we founded the EWG Action Fund, a 501(c)(4) organization that advocates on Capitol Hill for health-protective and subsidy-shifting policies. EWG specializes in providing useful resources (like Skin Deep and the Shoppers'

Guide to Pesticides in Produce) to consumers while simultaneously pushing for national policy change.

Reports:

No Silver Living: An Investigation into Bisphenol A in Canned Foods. 2010. Eating common canned foods is exposing consumers to levels of bisphenol A (BPA) equal to levels shown to cause health problems in laboratory animals, according to a new study released today by The National Work Group for Safe Markets, a coalition of public health and environmental health groups. The study, No Silver Lining, tested food from 50 cans from 19 US states and one Canadian province for BPA contamination. Over 90% of the cans tested had detectable levels of BPA, some at higher levels than have been detected in previous studies.

Full report at: http://www.ecocenter.org/press/releases/documents/NoSilverLiningBPAReport.pdf

FOOD, GROWING IT, FINDING IT AND EATING IT

Center for Science in the Public Interest. The Center for Science in the Public Interest (CSPI) is a consumer advocacy organization whose twin missions are to conduct innovative research and advocacy programs in health and nutrition, and to provide consumers with current, useful information about their health and well-being. Information on labeling laws as they affect restaurant menus and grocery store items. http://cspinet.org/index.html

Top Ten Resources for Local Food, reprinted with permission from *Pathways to Family Wellness* magazine.

Where to Find Local Food, Including Your Own Yard!
Have you taken time to explore your local foodshed? Have you taken the locavore's pledge below?
If not LOCALLY PRODUCED, then Organic.
If not ORGANIC, then Family farm.
If not FAMILY FARM, then Local business.
If not a LOCAL BUSINESS, then Fair Trade.

The term "foodshed" was used almost 80 years ago in a book entitled *How Great Cities Are Fed*, 1929, to describe the flow of food from producer to consumer. Eight decades later, the term is now used to describe a food system that connects local producers with local consumers. This summer, explore and support your local foodshed with the help of these Top Ten Local Food Resources. In this list you will find ways to connect, reasons to connect, how to preserve the bounty, tools for making sustainable food choices on the spot with iPhone apps, and how your local foodshed can begin in your own backyard with edible landscaping tips!

1. Local Harvest helps consumers learn about the various ways farmers get their food to market, whether through CSAs, farmer's markets, pick-your-own, or co-ops, and then provides a national listing of these local food outlets. Just enter your zip code to find local food outlets near you. Local Harvest also lists produce protected by the Ark of Taste, a Slow Food project that documents endangered varieties, like Deer Tongue lettuces! localharvest.org.

2. The Sustainable Table is home to the Eat Well Guide and the award-winning Meatrix movies. The Eat Well Guide is a free, online directory of sustainably-raised meat, poultry, dairy and eggs from farms, stores, restaurants, Bed and Breakfasts and other outlets in the United States and Canada. Consumers enter their zip or postal code to find wholesome products available locally or when traveling. sustainabletable.org

3. The Eat Local Challenge is a place to find inspiration and resources when the intention to eat local foods feels like an overwhelming commitment to conscious living. EatLocalChallenge.com is a group blog written by authors who are interested in the benefits of eating food grown and produced in their local foodshed. Spanning the United States, the group is committed to challenging themselves to eat mainly local food which means mastering the art of seasonal eating. Read their stories and recipes and share your own. eatlocalchallenge.com

4. The Weston A. Price Foundation is lead by president, Sally Fallon Morell, and her seminal work, *Nourishing Traditions: The Cookbook that Challenges Politically Correct Nutrition.* This well-researched, thought-provoking guide to traditional foods contains a startling message: Animal fats and cholesterol are not villains but vital factors in the diet, necessary for normal growth, proper function of the brain and nervous system, protection from disease and optimum energy levels. Start or find a local Weston Price Chapter for support and resources for local grass-fed meats. westonaprice.org.

5. Slow Food is an international movement founded in Italy in 1986 to preserve traditional and regional cuisine and promote farming of plants, seeds and livestock characteristics of the

local ecosystem. Slow Food USA is a non-profit organization working to create a just and sustainable food system. Slow Food USA has 225 volunteer-led chapters across the country, representing more than 150,000 members and advocates. The organization creates youth programs to bring the values of eating local, sustainable and just food to schools and campuses; preserves and promotes vanishing foods and food traditions; and advocates for food and farming policy that is good for the public, good for farmers and workers, and good for the planet. Start or find a chapter at slowfoodusa.org.

6. Real Milk Campaign. A project of the Weston A. Price foundation, the Real Milk Campaign educates and provides resources for local food enthusiasts to enjoy "real milk", that is, raw whole milk from grass-fed cows. Real milk is produced under clean conditions and promptly refrigerated, contains many anti-microbial and immune-supporting components; but this protective system in raw milk can be overwhelmed, and the milk contaminated, in situations conducive to filth and disease. The Real Milk Campaign tells consumers they must know their farmer to enjoy "real milk" and its nutritional benefits. Local and state chapters of this campaign work in states to preserve or legalize real milk options. realmilk.com.

7. This Shopper's Guide To Pesticides iPhone App from the Environmental Working Group when scouring farmer's markets, this guide will let you know which produce to buy organic, and which conventionally-grown fruits and vegetables are okay if organic isn't available. You can also receive EWG's email updates, action alerts and environmental tips. Download the app for free. foodnews.org.

8. Do you want seafood to be a part of your sustainable food choices? At a time when the world's oceans are severely overfished, your seafood choices make a big difference. The Monterey Bay Aquarium's iPhone application brings the latest Seafood Watch recommendations directly to your iPhone or iPod touch. Search for seafood by region. montereybayaquarium.org/cr/SeafoodWatch/web/sfw_iPhone.aspx

9. Think you need forty acres and a mule to grow your own food? Think again! You local foodshed can begin in your own backyard with the wisdom and practical guidance from books like *Food Not Lawns: How To Turn Your Yard Into a Garden And Your Neighborhood Into A Community* and *The Complete Book of Edible Landscaping: Home Landscaping With Edible Plants and Resource-Saving Techniques.* Both available online at Amazon.com. To start a local chapter of Food Not Lawns, visit them at foodnotlawns.net.

10. Now that you have discovered the treasures of your local foodshed, how will you preserve it for winter months? Learn the lost arts of storing the harvest from the National Center for Home Food Preservation. Learn to keep nutrient-dense, whole food for your family year round with information on canning or freezing vegetables and fruits, which dehydrators to use for making fruit leathers, sun drying or vine drying, and specialty crafts like making meat jerkies and leathers. uga.edu/nchfp.

This Top Ten Local Foodshed Resource List is reprinted with permission from *Pathways to Family Wellness* magazine. www. pathwaystofamilywellness.com.

APPENDIX:

Diet Of Clyde Vaughan

3,300 calories days
Insulin units will be multiplied by a 1.3 factor by insulin pump

MEATS

ITEM .... *UNITS OF INSULIN*

Palm hand size (5 oz).. 4 1/2 units
Pork .... 4 1/2 units
Tenderlion .... 4 1/2 units
Hamburger .... 4 1/2 units
Steak.. 4 1/2 units
Bar-b-que pork (sugar free sauce) .... 4 1/2 units
Fried fish (1/2 lbs) ....8 units
Fried shrimp (8shrimp)... 10 units
(32 to a lbs)
Crab meat patty...9 units

SOUP

Progresso New England Clam Chowder 18.5 can .... 1/2 with 5 units
With crackers.. 4 1/2 units
Homemade vegetables soup with 5 crackers .... 8 units

VEGETABLES (HOME GROWN)

Usually 3 Tablespoons of vegetables

Spaghetti	8 units
Fried okra-1/2 c	3 1/2 units
Butterbeans	2 units
Corn on cob (8 inches)	2 1/2 units
Crowder peas	2 units
Can garden peas	2 units
Broccoli (1/2 cup)	2 units
Mac & cheese (1/2 cup)	2 units
Cole slaw/mayo (1/2 cup)	2 units
Potato salad (1/2c)	-2 units
Unsweeted applesauce (1/2 c. with Splenda)	2 units
Beets (4-5 slices)	3 units
Frozen French fries (15 fries)	4 units

FRUITS

Apples (large)	7 units
California orange (navel)	7 units
Raisins (1.5 oz snack box)	7 units

COOKIES, DESSERTS AND SNACKS

Always check serving size
Divide by 30 to get units of insulin needed.

Pies (with splenda) 1 slice	7 units
1 slice cake (2 3/4 inches)	7 units
Ice cream (two scoops, fat free)	6 units
Muffins	7 units

Jello (1/4 cup) with 3 TBSp Cream.............................2 1/2 units
Can (8.75 oz, no syrup) peaches .... 6 units
popcorn(slightly salted, small bag) .... 3 units
Granola(1 bar) .... 6 1/2 units
Five peanut butter Ritz crackers .... 6 ½ units

MISCELLANEOUS

Pear salad/cheese .... 3 units

SANDWICHES

NOTE: All bread has 5% sugar
1 slice bread .... 2.3 units
Ham sandwiches .... 5 units
Bologna .... 5 units
With cheese.. 7 units
Pimento cheese .... 5 units
Block cheese .... 4 units

SUBWAY SANDWICHES

VERY ACCURATE IN CALORIES, divide by 30 to give units
of insulin

RESTAURANT:

Eating in restaurants requires at least three trips to solve the correct units to maintain blood glucose levels, eating identical din-
ners each time.

Shirley Shares Some of Her Southern Recipes:

PORK Bar-B-Q

1 3-4 lbs pork loin roast OR tenderloin
1 TBSP lemon juice
1/4 cup vinegar
1/2 cup BBQ sauce (Kraft)
1 – 8 oz can tomato sauce
3 TBSP brown sugar
2 TSP liquid smoke (optional)
Red and black pepper to taste

Mix and pour over pork roast. Cook in crock pot on low for eight to 10 hours. Pull apart with fork, serve on bun with slaw. (Make plenty for freezing)

CORNMEAL MUFFINS
(yield: 4 muffins)

2 TBSP Splenda
4 TSP vegetable oil
1 egg beaten
2 TBSP milk
1/4 cup cornmeal
1/4 cup all purpose flour
1/2 teaspoon baking powder

In a bowl, combine sugar, oil, egg and milk; mix well. In another bowl, combine dry ingredients; stir in Splenda mixture just until moistened. Pour into four muffin cups which have been lined with nonstick cooking spray.

BAKE at 400 for 15-18 minutes, until lightly brown

BRAN MUFFINS
- with nuts & raisins

1 1/3 cup all-purpose flour
1/2 cup Splenda OR 1/4 cup sugar (or less) & 1/4 cup Splenda
1 TBSP baking powder
1 1/2 cups Kellogg's ALL BRAN (40% Fiber) cereal
1 cup milk
1 egg
1/3 cup shortening (OR UNSWEETEND APPLESAUCE)

Stir together flour, Splenda, baking powder. Set aside In a large mixing bowl, combine all bran cereal and milk let set, about 2 min. until cereal is soften.

ALSO: ADD —- Apple pie spices (or cinnamon, nutmeg, pumpkin) any spices to your taste. I sometime use orange zest for flavor, about 1 teaspoon or so.

Add egg and shortening or applesauce (which I use).Mix well, and then add to flour mixture stirring only until combined.

Add nuts (walnuts, pecans etc.) and the raisins—to taste
Portion evenly into twelve 2 1/2 inch muffin pan coated with cooking spray.

BAKE at 400 degrees about 15-20 minutes, UNTIL lightly browned

YIELD: 12 MUFFINS

LEMON MERENGE PIE

1 1/4 CUPS WATER
1 CUP (1/2 cup Splenda; 1/2 or less sugar)
1 TBSP butter or margarine
1/3 cup cornstarch
3 TBPS cold water
3 eggs, separated (at room temperature
2 TBSP milk
6 TBSP lemon juice
1 TSP grated lemon rid
1 BAKED 8-inch pastry shell
6 TBSP (3 TBSP sugar; 3 TBSP Splenda)
1 TSP lemon juice

Combine water, sugar and butter in a heavy saucepan. Cook over medium heat until sugar is dissolved, stirring constantly. Dissolve cornstarch in cold water and to hot mixture, stirring constantly. Cook over medium heat until mixture is thickened and transparent (about five minutes.)

Beat egg yolks with milk; stir a small amount of hot mixture into yolks. Add yolk mixture to hot mixture in sauce pan stirring constantly. Cook two minutes longer, stirring constantly. Remove from heat and stir in six tablespoons lemon juice and lemon rind; cool slightly and spoon into pastry shell. Beat egg whites until soft peaks form; gradually add 6 tablespoons sugar and one teaspoon lemon juice, beating until stiff peaks form and sugar is dissolved.

Spread meringue over filling, making sure edges are sealed. Bake at 350 for 12 to 15 minutes or until golden brown. Yield: One eight inch pie.

More Tips from Clyde

HOW TO RECOGNIZE AND CORRECT BLOOD GLUCOSE HIGHS AND LOWS:

For Lows:

For me, and you might be different, I recognize my blood glucose lows by symptoms of increased hunger, lights become brighter, like television and lamps, and outside lights become hazy, and heavy perspiration. If I am going from the inside to the outside of the house, I might see floating clouds in this state. One aspect of a low blood sugar that is dangerous, of many, is that my eyes are unable to read the meter or pump, so I try not to let the first signs of a low go for more than a few seconds. I also learned the hard way (as in I ended up in the hospital) that when I have a low, I need to wait at least 40 minutes before returning to work in the garden, after adjusting my blood glucose with the following tricks:

FOOD INCREASE	BG UNITS
1 ounce of Coke	25
1 fun size snickers	15
1 orange slice	50
9 Hersey Kisses	3

The blood glucose highs aren't hard to recognize when they come on as Shirley says that is when I am a "pain in the ass." Symptoms of blood glucose highs for me are dizziness, shaking, loss of concentration, high blood pressure, for example, my blood pressure will be 244/108 if my blood glucose is over 400. And of course, Shirley's favorite, MOOD SWINGS.

For Highs:

If my blood glucose is 250 and blood glucose pump set point is 130, and one units of insulin lowers the blood glucose by 30 points, then the formula for lowering is:

(250-130) divided by 30 = number of units of insulin needed to adjust blood glucose to 130.

After the injection of insulin, a recheck at 45 minutes is important to see how well you did.

On Enzymes:

All TP survivors will have to take enzymes capsules for digestion of food. In the beginning, I used three different capsules successfully, until we went into the donut hole with our Medicare coverage. Then I was switched to two types of capsules manufactured in Italy - which caused lots of problems. The cost of the Italian enzymes was $1,000 or $1,300 for three months. When I am not in the donut hole, I use Ultrase, as there is no stomach pain, gas, and normal stool, color and odor as with the Italian brands. The cost of Ultrase, which is manufactured in USA, is $154 for three months. Currently the FDA is re-pricing some of these medications. Here is my guide for knowing how many enzymes to take with insulin units:

Units Of Insulin	Number Of Capsules
6 units of insulin	1
10 units of insulin	2
15 units of insulin	3
20 units of insulin	4
25 units of insulin	5

Insulin Ineffectiveness:

With my five and a half years of experience, I have found a host of environmental elements, foods and medicines which cause the insulin to lose its effectiveness and blood glucose management to be more difficult. Listed below are the ones I know from logging their effects, prevent insulin from working efficiently. The short list is:

- cigarettes
- wood smoke
- all narcotic (can take ibuprofen every four hours with little problems)
- prednisone
- mushrooms
- paint fumes

CITATIONS

INTRODUCTION

1 Estimates of Health-Care Associated Infections. Centers for Disease Control. www.cdc.gov/ncidod/dhqp/hai.html.

2 Phone Interview. Centers for Disease Control and Prevention and the National Center for Health Statistics, Media Officers, May 2, 2010.

3 Total pancreatectomy: Indications, different timing, and perioperative and long-term outcomes. Crippa S, Tamburrino D, Partelli S, Salvia R, Germenia S, Bassi C, Pederzoli P, Falconi M. Department of Surgery, Chirurgia Generale B - Pancreas Unit, Policlinico GB Rossi, University of Verona, Verona, Italy. Appearing ahead of print publication on May 20, 2010, online at PubMed. http://www.ncbi.nlm.nih.gov/pubmed/20494386.

4 Pancreatic Cancers Use Fructose, Common in a Western Diet, to Fuel Growth. Press Release. Heaney, Andrew, MD, PhD. Jonsson Comprehensive Cancer Center, University of California at Los Angeles. August 3, 2010. http://www.cancer.ucla.edu/Index.aspx?page=644&recordid=385&returnURL=/index.aspx

5 Diabetes epidemic out of control. Press Release. December 4, 2006. International Diabetes Federation. http://www.idf.org/diabetes-epidemic-out-control

6   Betsy Hilfiger's Close Call: An Unexpected Pancreatectomy. Patient Spotlights, The Pancreas Center, Columbia University. http://www.columbiasurgery.org/pancreas/guide_spotlights_ hilfiger.html

7   Native Americans embrace tradition to defeat diabetes. Marcus, Mary Brophy. USA Today. June 24, 2010. http://www. usatoday.com/news/health/2010-06-24-diabetestribes24_ ST_N.htm?csp=34news&utm_source=feedburner&utm_ medium=feed&utm_campaign=Feed:+usatoda y-NewsTopStories+(News+-+Top+Stories)

CHAPTER ONE: HOW I LOST MY PANCREAS, AND OUR DREAM OF PEACE

1   Estimates of Health-Care Associated Infections. Centers for Disease Control. www.cdc.gov/ncidod/dhqp/hai.html.

2   Think Like A Pancreas: A Practical Guide to Managing Diabetes with Insulin. Gary Scheiner, MS, CDE. Da Capo Press, Cambridge, MA. 2004.

CHAPTER TWO: BEYOND BRITTLE: TAKING INVENTORY, SEEKING PERSPECTIVE

1   Nicholson, William. American Edition of the British Encyclopedia or, Dictionary of Arts and Sciences; comprising an accurate and popular view of the present improved state of human knowledge, Volume 3. Mitchell, Ames and White. Philadelphia. 1819. Digitized by Google. http://

books.google.com/books?id=vHQaAQAAIAAJ&printsec=fr
ontcover&dq=American+Edition+of+the+British+Encyclope
dia&source=bl&ots=YhWjoiTAgZ&sig=4m5ajwHMbGRIc
ikFERVWooxaV-g&hl=en&ei=0gaFTPO8E4aWsgOSoKz
3Bw&sa=X&oi=book_result&ct=result&resnum=1&sqi=2&
ved=0CBcQ6AEwAA#v=onepage&q&f=false

2   Johnson, I.S. "Human insulin from recombinant DNA technology." Science Magazine. February 1983: Vol. 219. no.
4585, pp. 632 – 637. http://www.sciencemag.org/cgi/content/
abstract/219/4585/632

3   Richter B, Neises G. "'Human' insulin versus animal insulin
in people with diabetes mellitus." Department of Metabolic
Diseases and Nutrition, Heinrich-Heine University of
Duesseldorf, Moorenstr. 5, Duesseldorf, Germany. Cochrane
Database Syst Rev. 2005;(1):CD003816. http://www.ncbi.
nlm.nih.gov/pubmed/12917989

4   Insulin analog. Wikipedia, the Free Encyclopedia. March
2010. http://en.wikipedia.org/wiki/Insulin_analog

5   American Diabetes Association website. www.diabetes.org.

6   History of Diabetes. The Medical News. http://www.news-
medical.net/health/History-of-Diabetes.aspx

7   Diabetes Mellitus. Wikipedia, the Free Encyclopedia. http://
en.wikipedia.org/wiki/Diabetes_mellitus

8   The History of Diabetes. Melissa Sattley. Diabetes Health
magazine. November 1996. http://www.diabeteshealth.com/
read/2008/12/17/715/the-history-of-diabetes/

9   FDA Urged to Tighten Glucose Meter Standards. Kate Traynor.
American Society of Health-System Pharmacists. May
1, 2010. http://www.ashp.org/import/news/HealthSystem
PharmacyNews/newsarticle.aspx?id=3320

10 Accuracy of the GlucoWatch G2 Biographer and the Continuous Glucose Monitoring System During Hypoglycemia: Experience of the Diabetes Research in Children Network. Diabetes Care. American Diabetes Association. Vol. 27 No. 3, 722-726. March 2004. http://care.diabetesjournals.org/content/27/3/722.short

11 Glucophone. http://healthpia.us/.

12 The Glucowatch, glugophones, and other continuous automatic blood testers. Diabetes Recipes: Menu's, Meal's, and lifestyle advice for diabetics. http://diabetes-recipes.org/2008/12/05/the-glucowatch-continuous-blood-testing-for-diabetics/

13 The Stinging Cost of Glucose Test Strips. Diabetes Mine. October 9, 2007. http://www.diabetesmine.com/2007/10/the-stinging-co.html

14 American Diabetes Association website. www.diabetes.org.

15 Diabetes epidemic out of control. Press Release. December 4, 2006. International Diabetes Federation. http://www.idf.org/diabetes-epidemic-out-control

16 Total pancreatectomy: Indications, different timing, and perioperative and long-term outcomes. Crippa S, Tamburrino D, Partelli S, Salvia R, Germenia S, Bassi C, Pederzoli P, Falconi M. Department of Surgery, Chirurgia Generale B - Pancreas Unit, Policlinico GB Rossi, University of Verona, Verona, Italy. Appearing ahead of print publication on May 20, 2010, online at PubMed. http://www.ncbi.nlm.nih.gov/pubmed/20494386.

17 Is there still a role for total pancreatectomy? Müller MW, Friess H, Kleeff J, Dahmen R, Wagner M, Hinz U, Breisch-Girbig D, Ceyhan GO, Büchler MW. Department of General Surgery, University of Heidelberg, Heidelberg, Germany. Ann Surg. 2007 Dec;246(6):966-74; discussion 974-5. www.ncbi.nlm.nih.gov/pubmed/18043098

18 Phone interview. American Pancreatic Association. June 14, 2010. www.american-pancreatic-association.org.

CHAPTER THREE: I BECOME A LIVING MEDICAL EXPERIMENT AND SHIRLEY BECOMES A LOT OF THINGS

1 MiniMed Paradigm Insulin Pumps: Recall & Information. Defective Products. Free Advice ®. http://injury-law.freeadvice.com/defective_products/medtronic-minimed-paradigm-insulin-pump-recall.htm

2 Medtronic Insulin Pump Lawsuit: Recall of Quick-Set Infusions Sets for MiniMed Paradigm Insulin Pumps. Press release. Harvey Kirk. Saiontz and Kirk Law Firm. Pennsylvania. July 13, 2009. http://www.youhavealawyer.com/blog/2009/07/13/medtronic-insulin-pump-lawsuits/

3 FDA Public Health Notification: Potentially Fatal Errors with GDH-PQQ* Glucose Monitoring Technology. Press Release. US Food and Drug Administration. August 13, 2009. http://www.fda.gov/MedicalDevices/Safety/AlertsandNotices/PublicHealthNotifications/ucm176992.htm

CHAPTER FOUR: WHY WE SUED THE DOCTOR AND WHY WE LOST THE CASE

1 Grant Allows Creation of Nat Turner Rebellion Tour. Linda McNatt. The Virginian Pilot, via www.PilotOnline.com. August 4, 2010. http://hamptonroads.com/2010/08/grant-allows-creation-nat-turner-rebellion-tour

2   The Confessions of Nat Turner, The Leader of the Late
    Insurrection in Southampton, Virginia. Electronic Edition.
    Documenting the American South. Academic Affairs Library,
    University of North Carolina at Chapel Hill, 1999. http://
    docsouth.unc.edu/neh/turner/turner.html

CHAPTER FIVE: A CANARY IN A COALMINE

1   Burning News for Builders. Newsletter. University of
    Wisconsin–Extension, Center for Environment and Energy.
    www.c2p2online.com/documents/BuilderBurning.pdf.
2   Backyard Burning. Environmental Protection Agency website.
    www.epa.gov/wastes/nonhaz/municipal/backyard/index.htm
3   Facts on Trash Burning. Department of Environment
    Conservation. State of Vermont. www.dontburnvt.org/pdfs/
    TrashBurningFacts.pdf
4   Clearing the Air, Tools for Reducing Residential Garbage
    Burning. Compiled by the Western Lake Superior Sanitary
    District in partnership with the Minnesota Office of
    Environmental Assistance. Funded through a grant from the
    U.S. EPA Great Lakes National Program Office. www.wlssd.
    com/pdf/burning_reducing.pdf.
5   Backyard Trash Burning, Develop Awareness Materials.
    Environmental Protection Agency. www.epa.gov/air/com-
    munity/details/barrelburn.html
6   Clearing the Air, Tools for Reducing Residential Garbage
    Burning. Compiled by the Western Lake Superior Sanitary
    District in partnership with the Minnesota Office of
    Environmental Assistance. Funded through a grant from the

U.S. EPA Great Lakes National Program Office. www.wlssd. com/pdf/burning_reducing.pdf.

7   What is Body Burden? Coming Clean. Website. www. chemicalbodyburden.org/whatisbb.htm#

8   Top Ten Spring Cleaning Tips. Healthy Home Tips. EnvironmentalWorkingGroup.www.ewg.org/healthyhometips/ greencleaning.

9   Toxic America. CNN. http://www.cnn.com/SPECIALS/ 2010/toxic.america.

10 Safer Chemicals, Healthy Families. www.saferchemicals.org.

CHAPTER SIX: WHAT HAPPENED TO FOOD?

1   History of Peanuts. National Peanut Board. www.national-peanutboard.org/classroom-history.php

2   Ibid.

3   *Marker to Honor Man Who Invented the Peanut Picker.* By Merle Monahan. *Virginian Pilot.* May 29, 2008. http://findarticles. com/p/news-articles/virginian-pilot-ledger-star-norfolk/ mi_8014/is_20080529/marker-honor-invented-peanut-picker/ ai_n41403203/

4.   History of Peanuts. National Peanut Board. www.national-peanutboard.org/classroom-history.php

5   Pirog, Rich, and Andrew Benjamin. "Checking the Food Odometer: Comparing Food Miles for Local Versus Conventional Produce Sales in Iowa Institutions." Leopold Center for Sustainable Agriculture, July 2003.

6   *Pancreatic Cancers Use Fructose, Common in a Western Diet, to Fuel Growth.* Press Release. Heaney, Andrew, MD,

PhD. Jonsson Comprehensive Cancer Center, University of California at Los Angeles. August 3, 2010.http://www.cancer.ucla.edu/Index.aspx?page=644&recordid=385&return URL=/index.aspx

7 Food, Inc. www.foodincmovie.com.

8 A S.A.D. Lifestyle. Dr. Jeffrey S. McCombs. Huffington Post. November 17, 2008. http://www.huffingtonpost.com/dr-jeffrey-mccombs/a-sad-lifestyle_b_144395.html

9 Update on Bisphenol A for Use in Food Contact Applications: January 2010. Press Release. US Food and Drug Administration. www.fda.gov/NewsEvents/PublicHealthFocus/ucm197739.htm.

10 No Silver Lining. Contaminated Without Consent. http://contaminatedwithoutconsent.org/nosilverlining.php

CHAPTER SEVEN: AM I CRAZY?

1 Press release. "ADA MEETING: Diabetes and Depression Enhance Each Other's Severity and Cost." June 21, 1999. Doctor's Guide, Global Edition. http://www.pslgroup.com/dg/10b2ee.htm

2 "Number of Americans Taking Anti-Depressants Doubles." Szabo, Liz. USA Today. August 4, 2009. http://www.usatoday.com/news/health/2009-08-03-antidepressants_N.htm

CHAPTER EIGHT: THE PLAN

1 "5 Foods Its Cheaper to Grow." Sally Herigstad. MSN Money. http://articles.moneycentral.msn.com/SavingandDebt/SaveMoney/5FoodsItsCheaperToGrow.aspx

2   The Value of Growing Your Own Food. People Putting Food First #20. The Institute for Food and Development Policy. October 24, 2008. http://www.foodfirst.org/en/node/2290

3   Victory Gardens. Farming in the 1940s. Wessels Living History Farm. York, Nebraska.http://www.livinghistoryfarm. org/farminginthe40s/crops_02.html

4   Ibid.

5   *Native Americans embrace tradition to defeat diabetes.* Marcus, Mary Brophy. *USA Today.* June 24, 2010. http://www.usa-today.com/news/health/2010-06-24-diabetestribes24_ ST_N.htm?csp=34news&utm_source=feedburner&utm_ medium=feed&utm_campaign=Feed:+usatoda y-NewsTopStories+(News+-+Top+Stories)

CHAPTER NINE: CARING FOR THE CAREGIVER

1   Center for Science in the Public Interest website. Food Labeling. http://cspinet.org/new/200905141.html

2   Catching Up With Dale Evans. David Mendosa. *Diabetes Forecast.* March 2000, pages 76-78. www.mendosa.com/evans.htm

CHAPTER TEN: LIVING WITHOUT A PANCREAS

1   *Betsy Hilfiger's Close Call: An Unexpected Pancreatectomy.* Patient Spotlights, The Pancreas Center, Columbia University. http://www.columbiasurgery.org/pancreas/guide_spotlights_ hilfiger.html

2   Detecting a Cure. Kristi Birch. Johns Hopkins magazine. July 7, 2010 http://www.jhu.edu/jhumag/0405web/cancer.html

3   The President's Cancer Panel Report: "Reducing Environmental Cancer Risk: What We Can Do Now". May 18, 2010. http://www.healthandenvironment.org/partnership_calls/7309

4   Scoping Out Pancreatic Cancers Precursors. Johns Hopkins Gastroenterology and Hepatology. *Inside Tract*. Spring 2006.

5   Phone Interview. Joann Rodgers. Senior Advisor, Science, Crisis and Executive Communications to the to the Senior Director for Strategic Communications. Johns Hopkins. June 14, 2010.

6   Whipple Operation website. Center for Pancreatic and Biliary Diseases. University of Southern California, Department of Surgery.   http://www.surgery.usc.edu/divisions/tumor/pancreasdiseases/web%20pages/pancreas%20resection/whipple%20operation.html

7   Kidney and Pancreas Transplant Center website.   Cedars-Sinai Medical Center.   http://www.cedars-sinai.edu/Patients/Programs-and-Services/Kidney-and-Pancreas-Transplant-Center/.

8   "Current status of pancreatic islet Transplantation." Shaheed Merani and A. M. James Shapiro. Clinical Science (2006) 110, 611–625. Great Britian. http://www.clinsci.org/cs/110/0611/1100611.pdf

9   Pancreatectomy and Auto-Islet Transplant. Schulze Diabetes Institute, University of Minnesota. Website.http://www.diabetes.umn.edu/learnpancreatitis/treatmentspancreatitis/pancreatectomy/home.html